EATING WELL
THROUGH CANCER

Easy Recipes & Tips to Guide You Through **Treatment** and **Cancer Prevention**

HOLLY CLEGG & GERALD MILETELLO, M.D.

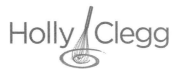

Library of Congress Control Number: 2016905711

ISBN-13   978-0-9815640-8-1
ISBN-10   0-9815640-8-9

Cover design and interior composition by Rikki Campbell Ogden / pixiedesign, llc
Edited by Lee Jackson, LDN, RD
Nutritional Analysis by Tammi Hancock, Hancock Nutrition

Available books by Holly Clegg:
    Holly Clegg's trim&TERRIFIC® KITCHEN 101
    Holly Clegg's trim&TERRIFIC® Too Hot in the Kitchen
    Holly Clegg's trim&TERRIFIC® Gulf Coast Favorites
    Holly Clegg trim&TERRIFIC® Diabetic Cooking
    Eating Well To Fight Arthritis
    Alimentándose bien durante el cáncer

Production and Manufacturing
Favorite Recipes Press
An imprint of
    FRP
P.O. Box 305142
Nashville, TN 37230
800-358-0560

On the back cover: Waldorf Salad, p. 18; Easy Potato Soup, p. 83; Lemon Bread, p. 15;
Butternut Squash, Black Bean, and Feta Enchiladas, p. 73

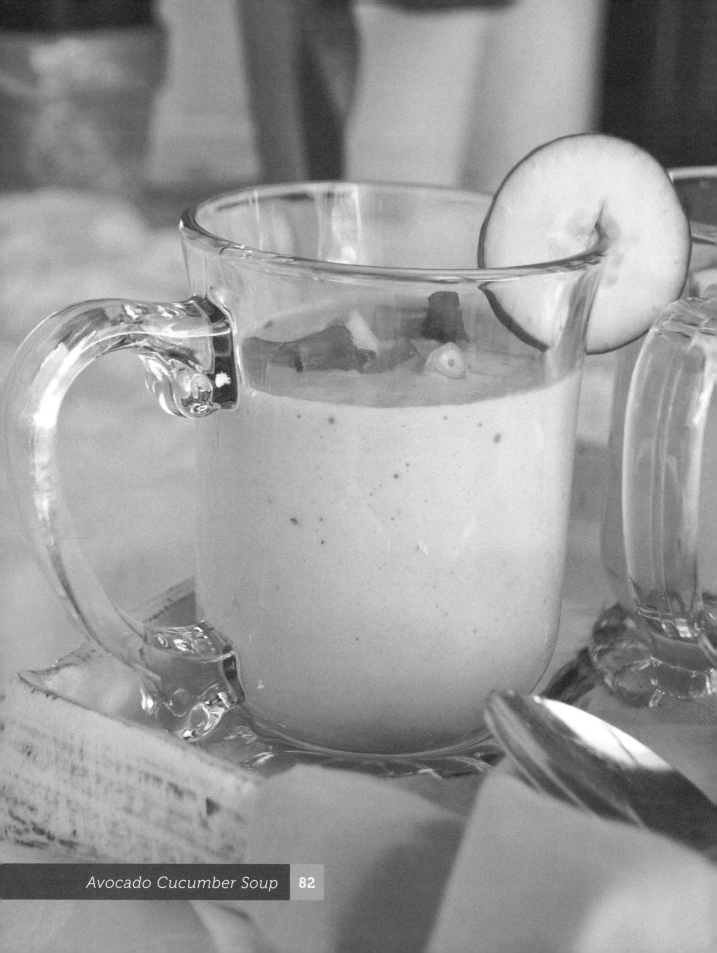

TABLE OF CONTENTS

· ·

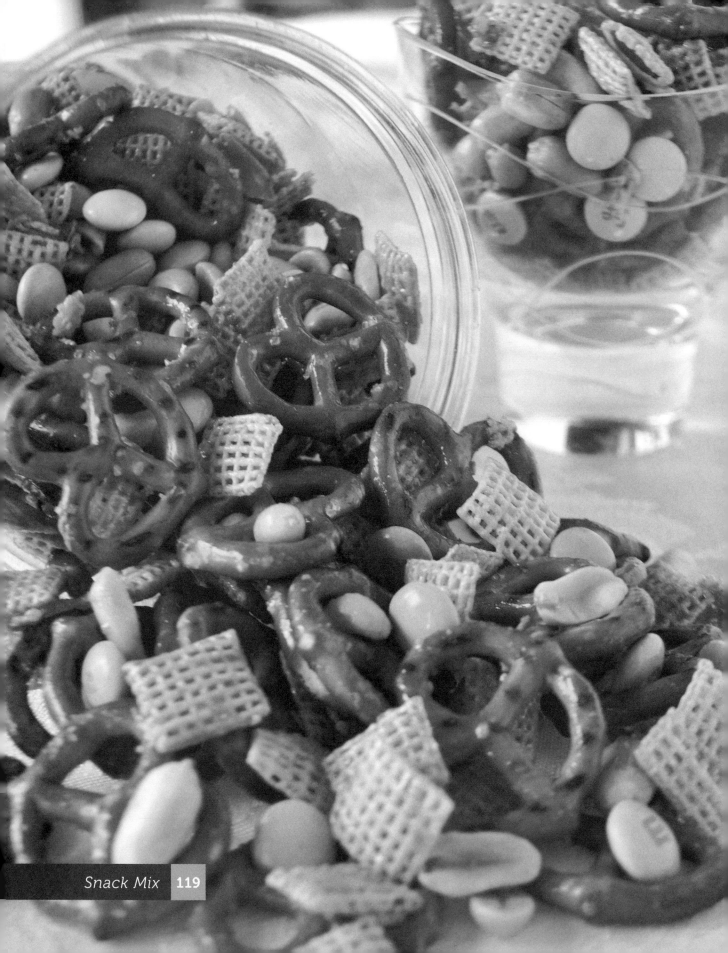

A NOTE FROM HOLLY

. . . .

The first edition of *Eating Well Through Cancer* came out in 2001 and was updated in 2006. Still one of the best-selling cancer cookbooks, I felt it was time to update and expand the cookbook with a fifteen year anniversary edition. As author of the *trim&TERRIFIC®* cookbook series, and my more health focused Eating Well series, I have sold over 1 million cookbooks! My hope is that these easy, healthy everyday cookbooks have helped people during challenging times and to lead an overall healthier lifestyle.

Years ago, Dr. Miletello pointed out to me that one of the most often asked questions by cancer patients was, "What can I eat?" Because of my love of food, this cancer cookbook was an opportunity for me to use my expertise in recipe development to create appropriate and best tolerated food addressing the side effects of cancer treatment. PEOPLE WITH CANCER STILL NEED TO EAT!

My challenge was to provide appealing EASY recipes that ease specific side effects during treatment. The chapters are organized into different side effects with approachable simple, nourishing recipes using familiar ingredients, but with an awareness of what a person can eat at each stage of treatment.

This book became very personal as my father was diagnosed with larynx cancer and had to undergo treatment. I better understood the everyday challenges he faced with eating. Fifteen years later, he speaks with an artificial larynx and still looks forward to my cooking.

We hope our book will help guide you through treatment, support the caregiver and be a recipe resource for a healthy kitchen for cancer prevention. Eating is a necessity and we hope these simple, super-satisfying recipes will make treatment a little easier with the comfort of food.

A NOTE FROM GERALD MILETELLO, MD

Cancer is an uncontrolled growth of cells that destroys the function of normal cells. Cancer can involve one organ of the body or every organ, including the blood. Once your treatment for cancer begins, you will likely notice a change in your appetite and your sense of taste and smell. The changes are secondary to normal cells being destroyed, as well as cancer cells. The goal of cancer treatment is to destroy the cancer cells and allow the good cells to flourish.

The loss of appetite, called anorexia, is one of the most common side-effects of chemotherapy. Trying to maintain adequate calorie intake during this time can be very difficult for the patient or caregiver who is trying to prepare food. You have to maintain your nutrition in order to maintain your health and strength to enable you to fight the cancer. Certain foods that you once loved may no longer appeal to you. Your taste and cravings may change from day to day and hour to hour. You may also develop side effects from the treatment or from the medication.

We hope that we can offer suggestions for food and drinks that will appeal to you, as well as suggestions for foods that will assist in managing some of the side-effects of chemotherapy. Although no diet has been proven to prevent cancer, health authorities agree that a properly chosen diet can reduce the risk of developing certain cancers and can help you to fight cancer.

ABOUT THE BOOK

Freezer-friendly recipes that you can make ahead

Vegetarian recipes

Gluten-free recipes

Diabetic-friendly recipes that meet ADA guidelines

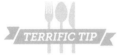

Short-cuts, options and tidbits about the recipes

Doc's tips for treatment

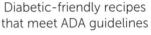
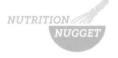

Nutritional information about ingredients used in the recipes

- Most recipes are *diabetic-friendly*, making this cookbook a great resource for people with diabetes or for those who strive for a healthier diet. Also, some of the drugs used to treat cancer may elevate your blood sugar.

- Each recipe includes the nutritional analysis and the diabetic exchange. The analysis is based on the larger serving. The nutritional analysis does not include any salt or pepper (since it is listed to taste) or any ingredient with "optional" after it.

- Low-sodium products are used throughout the book, but regular products may be substituted.

- As I tested these recipes on my family, I must emphasize that anyone who enjoys a healthier approach to cooking, with or without a health problem, will also enjoy this cookbook.

- It is important to note that you can use recipes from all chapters as many recipes fit in more than one category, just depending on how you feel.

- Good nutrition is essential to staying healthy and having the necessary energy for optimal quality of life.

- The recipes are for everyone, not only the cancer patient. The entire family can enjoy each and every one of these dishes.

MENUS

The menus are divided up into the chapter side effects, however, since all recipes are for a healthy lifestyle, you will find recipes from different chapters throughout the menus as most recipes fit in more than one chapter.

. . . .

1. DAY OF CHEMOTHERAPY

Morning of Chemotherapy
Applesauce Oatmeal | **80**
Egg in the Bread | **48**
Cheese Grits | **81**
Tea, Coffee, or Sports Drink

Evening of Chemotherapy
Easy Potato Soup | **83**
Toast
One Step Macaroni and Cheese | **21**
Sliced Turkey or Chicken Sandwiches
Peanut Butter and Jelly Sandwich
Nutritional Supplement Shake

Morning Following Chemotherapy
Tea
Toast
Gingerbread Muffins | **45**
Fresh Fruit with Yogurt
Smoothie (Chapter 7, p. 112)

Lunch 24 Hours Past Chemotherapy
Bread Pudding Florentine | **12**
Chicken, Barley, and Bow Tie Soup | **16**
Tuna Salad | **17**
Water

Dinner 24 Hours Past Chemotherapy
Simple Baked Chicken | **22**
Light and Lemon Angel Hair | **55**
Rice Pudding | **57**

Remember 6-8 cups of fluid per day

2. NEUTROPENIA

Breakfast
Oatmeal Banana Pancakes | **65**
Easy Cinnamon Rolls | **14**

Lunch
Roasted Chicken and Angel Hair | **23**
Cream Cheese Bread Pudding | **91**

Dinner
Oven Fried Crunchy Chicken | **53**
One Step Macaroni and Cheese | **21**
. . . . .
Pulled Pork Sandwich (no condiments) | **159**
Peanut Butter Cookies | **197**
. . . . .
Spinach Artichoke Dip (use as side) | **89**
Spicy Baked Fish | **37**
Baked Peach Delight | **38**

Snacks
Mini Cheese Pizzas (no veggies) | **130**
Snack Mix | **119**
Parmesan Pitas | **126**

3. NAUSEA

Breakfast
Egg in the Bread | **48**
Scrambled Egg Muffin | **49**
Applesauce
Easy Banana Bread, Toasted | **46**

Lunch
Roasted Chicken Soup with Rice | **50**
Banana Pudding | **57**

Dinner

Glazed Ginger Chicken | **52**
Couscous and Edamame | **56**
. . . . .
Chicken Scallopini | **51**
Light and Lemon Angel Hair | **55**
Rice Noodle Medley | **54**
Sweet Potato Biscuits | **26**

Snacks

Gingerbread Muffins | **45**
Rice Pudding | **57**

4. HIGH FIBER

Breakfast

Honey Bran Muffins | **75**
Harvest Granola | **117**
Fresh Fruit

Lunch

Barley Soup | **62**
Butternut Squash, Black Bean and
   Feta Enchiladas | **73**

Salad Medley

Black Bean and Corn Salad | **66**
Chicken Taco Rice Salad | **67**
Waldorf Salad | **18**

Dinner

Roasted Seasoned Salmon | **36**
Southwestern Baked Sweet Potatoes | **72**
Brussels Sprouts, Tomato and
   Feta Salad | **169**
. . . . .
Cuban Pork and Black Beans | **103**
Quick Spanish Rice | **194**
. . . . .
Pulled Chicken | **33**
Baked Beans | **68**
Southwestern Sweet Potato Salad | **153**

Snacks

Guacamame, Fresh Vegetables | **122**
Meaty Mediterranean Pita Nachos | **127**

5. SORE MOUTH

Breakfast

Cheese Grits | **81**
Bread Pudding Florentine | **12**
Applesauce Oatmeal | **80**
Soft fruits such as watermelon, papaya

Lunch

Avocado Cucumber Soup | **82**
Cheese Quesadillas | **130**
Pistachio Pudding with Chocolate Sauce | **92**

Dinner

Simple Baked Chicken | **22**
(chicken cut into small pieces)
Creamed Double Potatoes | **87**
Watermelon and Cantaloupe Salad | **85**
. . . . .
Chicken Pot Pie | **86**
(chicken and vegetables cut into small pieces)
Rice Pudding | **57**
. . . . .
Chicken and Dumplings | **24**
(chicken cut into small pieces, cook carrots until soft)
Quick Flan | **90**

Snacks

Guacamame | **122**
Smoothie (Chapter 7, p. 112)

6. HIGH CALORIE-HIGH PROTEIN

Breakfast

Tasty Tropical Smoothie | **135**
Shrimp and Peppers with Cheese Grits | **98**
Mexican Breakfast Casserole | **142**

Lunch

Black Bean Soup | **61**
Pulled Pork Sandwich | **159**
Southwestern Sweet Potato Salad | **153**
Waldorf Salad | **18**
. . . . .
Tuna with Broccoli and White Bean Pasta | **106**
Watermelon and Tomato Salad | **167**
Peanut Butter Cookies | **197**

continued on next page

DAY OF CHEMOTHERAPY

Easier to tolerate and lighter recipes to help boost
your immune system for strength and energy.

. . . .

Is there a certain time of day that is better for eating?

I only like two foods.

I cannot eat, but I can drink.

Nothing tastes good.

How do I overcome weight loss?

How do I prepare my pantry?

. . . .

Not all treatments will cause nausea, vomiting or loss of appetite. The acute side effects, such as nausea, are caused by the destruction of rapidly dividing cells lining the gastrointestinal tract. This is one of the primary causes for the loss of appetite, nausea, vomiting and sore mouth.

I recommend a low fat, light meal prior to your treatment, including foods such as cereal, toast, oatmeal, grits, fruit cocktail, peach or pear nectar. Twenty-four hours following your treatment, try liquids, soups, puddings or sandwiches. Try to avoid high fat, fried or greasy foods for the first twenty-four to forty-eight hours following treatment. If you find that only two foods appeal to you, then there is nothing wrong with eating those foods until you feel like expanding your diet. Water is essential. Eight to ten glasses of water per day are recommended. Supplements such as Boost are excellent choices if you only feel like drinking.

You may experience a sore or dry mouth as well as a total loss of appetite. This may require a little creativity on your part to keep your nutritional status on the positive side. You may find it impossible to eat three large meals per day. I recommend to you that you eat snacks daily. Six small meals instead of three large meals will increase your caloric intake. If your appetite does not improve, ask your doctor about an appetite stimulant such as megace 800mg per day × 30 days, then decrease to 400mg per day. The other option is Megace 40mg by mouth twice per day along with Marinol 2.5mg twice per day. Remember hydration is of utmost importance. Keep a glass of liquid available at all times. (Water with a slice of lemon, apple juice, carrot juice, cranberry juice, etc.).

Do not forget your mouth care protocol. This really will keep your mouth refreshed and decrease ulcer formation. Mix 1 teaspoon salt with 1 teaspoon baking soda in 1 quart water. Rinse and spit after each meal or at least four times per day. Mix fresh each morning using tap water.

Remember, your mouth will get better. The soreness normally clears within a few days. Food is medicine. You have to eat to get through these treatments and back to normal. Rinsing with Ulcerease, Viscous Xylocaine, or Cephacol lozenges may soothe your mouth before a meal.

FOR A SORE MOUTH

- Avoid any food that may irritate your mouth. Includes oranges, lemons, tomato sauces, crackers and alcohol.

- Avoid hot or extremely cold foods since they tend to irritate your mouth.

- Foods at room temperature or slightly cool foods are much more soothing.

- Try cutting your food into small pieces.

- Cook food until tender or even try pureeing food with a food processor.

- Drinking with a straw will sometimes help liquids go down easier.

DAY OF CHEMOTHERAPY AND FOLLOWING TREATMENT TIPS

- Eat smaller portions more frequently. Drink fluids between meals instead of with food.

- Eat by the clock at regularly scheduled times. Your appetite signal may not be intact.

- Eat between meals with high-protein diet supplements, milkshakes, puddings, or nutritional drink supplements.

- Add extra protein to your diet by using fortified milk, yogurt, peanut butter, cheese and chopped hard boiled eggs.

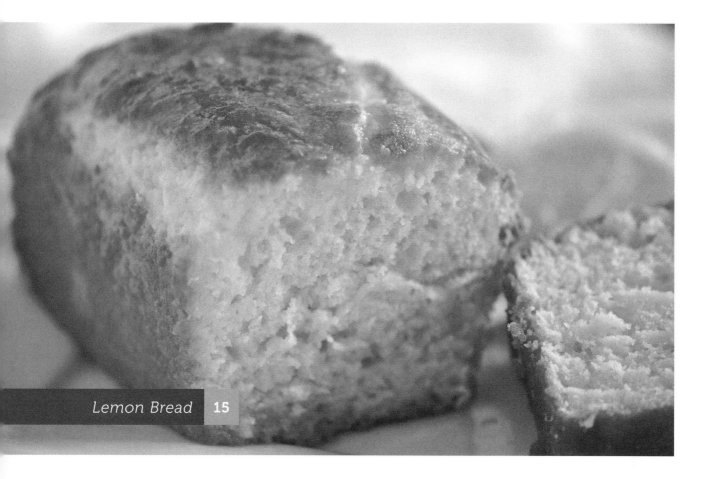

Lemon Bread 15

- Add cream or butter to soups, cooked cereals, and vegetables to increase calories. Add gravies and sauces to vegetables, meat, poultry and fish until weight loss is no longer a problem.

- Try to avoid empty calories: make snacks rich in protein and calories as these help the body heal.

- Try things to enhance smell, appearance, and texture of food. Be creative with desserts.

- Choose foods you like as long as you do not have dietary restrictions.

- Exercise approximately 30 minutes before meals to try to stimulate your appetite.

- Try to make mealtimes pleasant by eating with family or friends.

- Plan menus in advance. Have some food frozen and ready to heat and serve.

CHANGES IN FLAVOR

Cancer often affects the taste buds, commonly reducing the ability to taste sweetness. This changes the flavor of sweets, desserts, fruits and vegetables.

Some people experience an unusual dislike for certain foods, flavors, or odors. This develops when unpleasant symptoms are tied to a food recently eaten. Save your favorite foods for times when you feel well or eat your favorite food anytime (if you feel like a breakfast snack in the middle of the night, do it).

- Try not to eat one to two hours before treatment or therapy.

- If you no longer enjoy beef or pork, you may find chicken, fish, eggs, milk products or legumes more appealing.

- Marinate meats or cook them with sauces or tomatoes to help improve the flavor.

- Meats that are cold or at room temperature may be more palatable.

- A third potential taste change is an increased liking for tart flavors. Adding lemon juice to foods may make them taste better. A cancer patient may enjoy grapefruit, cranberry, or other tart juices.

TIPS TO EASE AT-HOME COOKING

- Wash and dry lettuce and seal in plastic containers or a greens bag for easy use.

- Wash, cut up and store veggies to have ready for snacks or use in recipes.

- Raid the salad bar for cut up veggies for recipes or for ready-to-eat products.

- Shred cheese and store in zip top bags or buy shredded cheese.

- When chopping onion or garlic, chop more than needed and store in zip top bags in the freezer for later use or buy pre-chopped seasoning at the grocery.

- Double recipes to freeze for a later date or freeze leftovers.

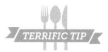

BREAD PUDDING FLORENTINE

This delicous make-ahead savory bread pudding makes a light breakfast-style recipe. Pop in a cold oven if using a glass dish when baking.

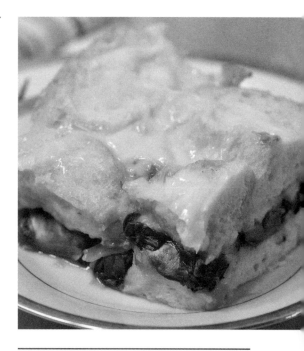

Half loaf French or Italian bread, cut into slices, divided
1/2 pound mushrooms, sliced
1 onion, chopped
1 teaspoon minced garlic
2 cups packed baby spinach
2 teaspoons all-purpose flour
Salt and pepper to taste
1 cup shredded reduced-fat Swiss cheese, divided
2 eggs
3 egg whites
1 1/2 cups skim milk
2 teaspoons Dijon mustard

1 Coat a 9×9×2-inch baking dish with nonstick cooking spray. Place half of the bread slices in prepared dish.

2 In large nonstick skillet coated with nonstick cooking spray, sauté mushrooms, onion, and garlic until tender. Add spinach, stirring until wilted, and add flour, stirring to mix well. Season to taste; set aside.

3 Spread spinach mixture over bread and sprinkle with 3/4 cup cheese. Top with remaining bread and remaining 1/4 cup cheese.

4 In bowl, whisk together eggs, egg whites, milk, and mustard. Pour egg mixture evenly over casserole, refrigerate 2 hours or overnight.

5 When ready to cook, preheat oven 350°F. Bake 40–50 minutes or until puffed and golden.

MAKES 7 (3/4-cup) servings

PREP TIME 15 minutes + refrigerate 2 hours

COOK TIME 50 minutes

TERRIFIC TIP

You can substitute 1 (10-ounce) box frozen chopped spinach, thawed and squeezed dry for fresh spinach. Adjust mushrooms and onions to your taste buds.

DOC'S NOTE

This is a great dish to try several days before your next cycle of treatment. Good source of vitamins and minerals.

NUTRITIONAL INFORMATION Calories 210, Calories from Fat 22%, Fat 5 g, Saturated Fat 2 g, Cholesterol 62 mg, Sodium 352 mg, Carbohydrates 26 g, Dietary Fiber 2 g, Total Sugars 6 g, Protein 16 g

DIABETIC EXCHANGES 1 starch, 1 fat, 1 lean meat, 2 vegetables

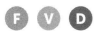

FLORENTINE ENGLISH MUFFINS

Creamed spinach and mozzarella on muffin halves make a quick breakfast. Top with fresh tomato slices, if desired.

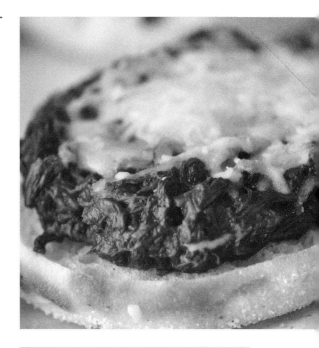

2 (10-ounce) packages frozen chopped spinach
1 tablespoon all-purpose flour
1 cup skim milk
Salt and pepper to taste
5 English muffins, cut in half
1 cup shredded part-skim mozzarella cheese

1 Cook spinach according to package directions, drain very well.

2 In nonstick pot, mix flour and milk over medium heat, stirring until thickened, about 5 minutes. Stir in spinach and season to taste.

3 Lay English muffin halves on baking sheet. Divide about 1/4 cup spinach mixture evenly on top of each muffin half. Sprinkle with mozzarella.

4 Preheat broiler. Place under broiler 1–2 minutes, or until cheese is melted and muffin begins to brown. Watch carefully.

MAKES 10 servings
PREP TIME 15 minutes
COOK TIME 5 minutes

TERRIFIC TIP

To freeze: Before cooking, wrap individually in freezer zip-top bags, label, and freeze.

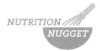

NUTRITION NUGGET

Did you know spinach is high in vitamin C? Vitamin C is an antioxidant and water-soluble vitamin that plays an important role in growth and tissue repair.

NUTRITIONAL INFORMATION Calories 123, Calories from Fat 19%, Fat 3 g, Saturated Fat 1 g, Cholesterol 8 mg, Sodium 227 mg, Carbohydrates 18 g, Dietary Fiber 2 g, Total Sugars 2 g, Protein 8 g

DIABETIC EXCHANGES 1/2 lean meat, 1 starch, 1 vegetable

EASY CINNAMON ROLLS

Keep canned biscuits handy to make this fast and fabulous treat for breakfast or a snack.

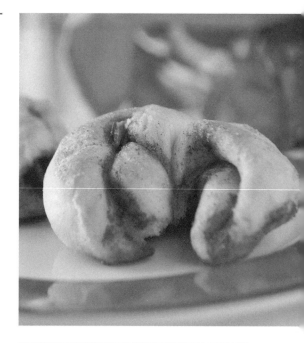

1 (10-biscuit) can refrigerated biscuits or whole-wheat biscuits
2 tablespoons butter
1 tablespoon sugar
1 teaspoon ground cinnamon
1/4 cup chopped pecans, optional

1 Preheat oven 425°F. Coat 15×10×1-inch baking pan with nonstick cooking spray.

2 Flatten each biscuit with your hand or rolling pin. Spread each biscuit with butter.

3 In small bowl, combine sugar and cinnamon together. Sprinkle cinnamon mixture on top of butter; sprinkle with pecans, if desired.

4 Roll up each biscuit like a cigar and form a circle by putting the ends together. Bake 8–10 minutes or until golden brown.

MAKES 10 rolls
PREP TIME 10 minutes
COOK TIME 10 minutes

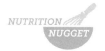

TERRIFIC TIP

Try using whole-wheat biscuits. Cinnamon rolls freeze to pop out for a quick snack.

· · · · · · · · · · · · · · · · · ·

NUTRITION NUGGET

Light, low-fat meals, especially breakfast foods seem to be the best tolerated of all foods while you are having chemotherapy.

NUTRITIONAL INFORMATION Calories 76, Calories from Fat 35%, Fat 3 g, Saturated Fat 1 g, Cholesterol 6 mg, Sodium 210 mg, Carbohydrates 11 g, Dietary Fiber 0 g, Total Sugars 3 g, Protein 1 g

DIABETIC EXCHANGES 1 starch, 1/2 fat

LEMON BREAD

This luscious lemon bread is my "go to" easy favorite. Make with or without the glaze but the glaze adds that sweet tartness in every bite.

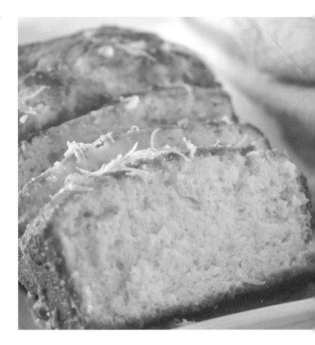

1 (8-ounce) package reduced-fat cream cheese
3/4 cup plus 2 tablespoons sugar, divided
2 eggs
1 tablespoon lemon extract
1 1/2 cups biscuit baking mix
2 tablespoons lemon juice

1 Preheat oven 350°F. Coat 9×5×3-inch nonstick loaf pan with nonstick cooking spray.

2 In large mixing bowl, mix together cream cheese and 3/4 cup sugar until light and fluffy. Beat in eggs and lemon extract.

3 Stir in baking mix just until blended. Transfer batter to prepared pan. Bake 40–50 minutes or until toothpick inserted comes out clean.

4 Immediately poke holes in 1-inch intervals on top of bread with toothpick. In microwave-safe dish, combine remaining 2 tablespoons sugar and lemon juice, heating until sugar is dissolved. Pour evenly over top of bread. Cool and slice.

MAKES 16 servings
PREP TIME 10 minutes
COOK TIME 45 minutes

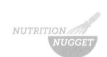

This recipe may also be made into muffins. Breads or muffins freeze well to pull out for an immediate snack or breakfast.

. . . .

NUTRITION
NUGGET

If you're experiencing taste changes, lemon flavoring may help reduce sour or bitter taste.

NUTRITIONAL INFORMATION Calories 132, Calories from Fat 30%, Fat 4 g, Saturated Fat 2 g, Cholesterol 33 mg, Sodium 201 mg, Carbohydrates 20 g, Dietary Fiber 0 g, Total Sugars 12 g, Protein 3 g

DIABETIC EXCHANGES 1 1/2 carbohydrate, 1 fat

CHICKEN, BARLEY, AND BOW TIE SOUP

A delicious one pot hearty version of a favorite remedy, chicken soup, with barley and pasta. This recipe makes a big pot to have throughout the week for an afternoon snack or light meal when you don't have an appetite.

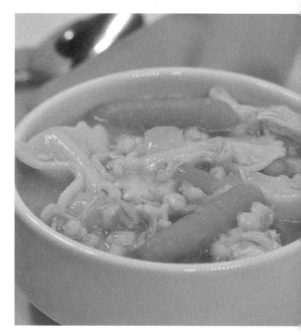

1 cup chopped celery
1 cup chopped onion
2 cups baby carrots
8 cups fat-free chicken broth
1/2 cup pearl barley
2 cups bow tie pasta (uncooked)
1/2 teaspoon dried basil leaves
2 cups skinless coarsely chopped rotisserie chicken
Salt and pepper to taste

1 In large nonstick pot coated with nonstick cooking spray, sauté celery, onion, and carrots, about 5–7 minutes. Add broth and barley. Bring to boil, reduce heat, cover, and cook about 20–30 minutes or until barley is done.

2 Meanwhile, cook pasta according to package directions; drain and set aside. When soup is done, add pasta, basil, and chicken. Season to taste. Heat 5 minutes.

MAKES 10 (1-cup) servings
PREP TIME 15 minutes
COOK TIME 30 minutes

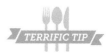

If experiencing taste changes, add extra seasonings as needed to perk up your taste buds. Serve soup in a mug and if temperature bothers you, serve only warm or room temperature.

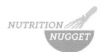

Barley is a whole grain and is high in fiber—adding great texture and taste to the soup. Barley may be left out for a plain chicken and noodle soup.

NUTRITIONAL INFORMATION Calories 186, Calories from Fat 10%, Fat 2 g, Saturated Fat 1 g, Cholesterol 28 mg, Sodium 137 mg, Carbohydrates 28 g, Dietary Fiber 3 g, Total Sugars 3 g, Protein 14 g

DIABETIC EXCHANGES 2 starch, 1 1/2 lean meat

TUNA SALAD

A light, fabulous tuna salad.

2 (6-ounce) cans solid white tuna, packed in water, drained
1 (11-ounce) can mandarin oranges, drained
1/4 pound sliced fresh mushrooms
1 (14-ounce) can quartered artichoke hearts, drained
1/2 cup sliced water chestnuts, drained
1/4 cup light mayonnaise
1/4 cup nonfat plain Greek yogurt
1 tablespoon lemon juice
2 teaspoons sugar
1 bunch green onions, chopped

1 In large bowl, carefully combine tuna, oranges, mushrooms, artichoke hearts, and water chestnuts.

2 In a medium bowl, combine mayonnaise, yogurt, lemon juice, sugar, and green onions to create a dressing.

3 Fold the dressing into the tuna mixture. Refrigerate until serving.

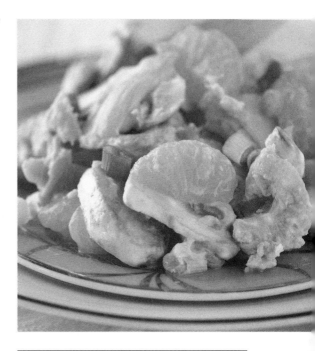

MAKES 8 servings
PREP TIME 15 minutes

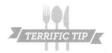
TERRIFIC TIP

Plan ahead to keep light, quick meals on hand, such as this salad for a quick nutritious meal.

· · · · · · · · · · · · · · · · ·

DOC'S NOTE

Tart flavors such as lemon and citrus may be extra palatable when not feeling well or if experiencing taste changes.

NUTRITIONAL INFORMATION Calories 108, Calories from Fat 14%, Fat 2 g, Saturated Fat 0 g, Cholesterol 19 mg, Sodium 324 mg, Carbohydrate 11 g, Dietary Fiber 3 g, Total Sugars 6 g, Protein 12 g

DIABETIC EXCHANGES 1 1/2 very lean meat, 2 vegetable

WALDORF SALAD

Apples, grapes, raisins and walnuts in a light citrus dressing keep this classic salad delicious while also being a great source of fiber, vitamins and minerals.

6 cups chopped apples (red and green)
2 stalks celery, chopped
1 cup red or green seedless grapes
1/2 cup chopped walnuts, toasted
1/2 cup raisins
1 cup nonfat plain yogurt
1/4 cup light mayonnaise
1/4 cup fresh orange juice

1 In large bowl combine apples, celery, grapes, walnuts, and raisins.

2 In another bowl, mix yogurt, mayonnaise, and orange juice. Toss with apple mixture and refrigerate until serving.

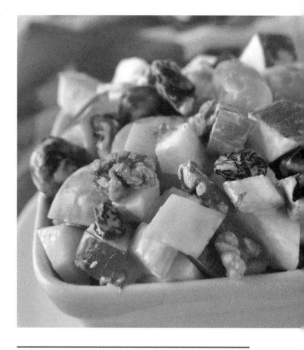

MAKES 10 (1-cup) servings

PREP TIME 15 minutes

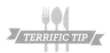

This is not only filled with fiber, but is very colorful and will surely stimulate your taste buds. For added calories, don't use fat-free products.

· · · · · · · · · · · · · · · · ·

DOC'S NOTE

If your appetite signal is off after chemotherapy, eat by the clock at regularly scheduled times.

NUTRITIONAL INFORMATION Calories 145, Calories from Fat 35%, Fat 5 g, Saturated Fat 1 g, Cholesterol 2 mg, Sodium 75 mg, Carbohydrates 24 g, Dietary Fiber 3 g, Total Sugars 18 g, Protein 3 g

DIABETIC EXCHANGES 1 1/2 fruit, 1 fat

OVEN BAKED RISOTTO

No time consuming stirring to whip up this scrumptious risotto recipe. Serve as a side or add additional ingredients to create an entrée. (Note: Only diabetic-friendly when served as side.)

2 tablespoons butter, melted
2 1/2 cups low-sodium fat-free chicken broth
1 cup Arborio rice
1 cup chopped onion
Salt and pepper to taste

1 Preheat oven 400 F°. In 13×9×2-inch baking dish, mix together butter, broth, rice, onion and season to taste.

2 Bake, covered, 35 minutes or until rice is done. Remove from oven and fluff rice with fork.

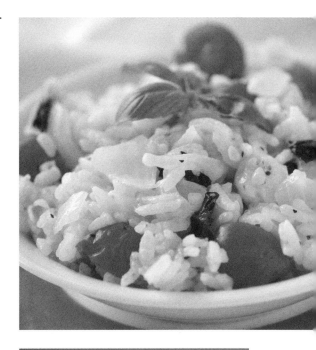

MAKES 5 (1-cup) entrees or 10 (1/2-cup) side servings

PREP TIME 5 minutes

COOK TIME 35 minutes

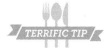

TERRIFIC TIP

For a heartier delicious option, after risotto is cooked, add fresh mozzarella, tomatoes, fresh basil and chicken.

· · · · · · · · · · · · · · · · ·

NUTRITION NUGGET

Arborio rice is often used to make risotto as it undergoes less milling, keeping more of its starch content, making it creamy in texture.

ENTRÉE NUTRITIONAL INFORMATION Calories 186, Calories from Fat 24%, Fat 5 g, Saturated Fat 3 g, Cholesterol 12 mg, Sodium 112 mg, Carbohydrates 32 g, Dietary Fiber 1 g, Total Sugars 2 g, Protein 3 g

DIABETIC EXCHANGES 2 starch, 1/2 fat

SIDE NUTRITIONAL INFORMATION Calories 93, Calories from Fat 24%, Fat 2 g, Saturated Fat 1 g, Cholesterol 6 mg, Sodium 56 mg, Carbohydrates 16 g, Dietary Fiber 1 g, Total Sugars 1 g, Protein 2 g

DIABETIC EXCHANGES 1 starch

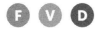

F V D

MAKES 6 (1-cup) servings

PREP TIME 5 minutes | **COOK TIME** 10 minutes

PERFECT PASTA

Parsley and garlic give simple angel hair pasta lots of flavor.

1 (12-ounce) package angel hair pasta
3 tablespoons olive oil
1 teaspoon minced garlic
2 tablespoons finely chopped parsley

1. Cook pasta according to directions on package.
   Drain and set aside.

2. In small pan, combine all remaining ingredients and sauté for few minutes. Toss with cooked pasta.

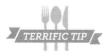

TERRIFIC TIP

Keep edamame in the freezer for a quick nutritious snack or to toss in recipes—like this pasta dish.

NUTRITIONAL INFORMATION Calories 271, Calories from Fat 26%, Fat 8 g, Saturated Fat 1 g, Cholesterol 0 mg, Sodium 5 mg, Carbohydrates 43 g, Dietary Fiber 1 g, Total Sugars 2 g, Protein 7 g

DIABETIC EXCHANGES 3 starch, 1 fat

F V D

MAKES 9 (3/4-cup) servings

PREP TIME 5 minutes | **COOK TIME** 15 minutes

LINGUINE FLORENTINE

Spinach, linguine and Parmesan team up for a light pasta side.

2 tablespoons olive oil
1 teaspoon minced garlic
6 cups baby spinach
1 (12-ounce) can evaporated skimmed milk
Salt and pepper to taste
1 (16-ounce) package linguine
1/3 cup grated Parmesan cheese

1. In large nonstick skillet, heat oil, add garlic and spinach. Cook, covered, until spinach is wilted, 3 minutes, stirring occasionally. Add milk, season to taste.

2. Meanwhile, prepare pasta according to package directions; drain. Toss with spinach; sprinkle with cheese.

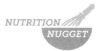

NUTRITION **NUGGET**

Spinach is full of nutrition made known by its vibrant rich green color—concentrated in phytonutrients and flavonoids, offering healthy antioxidant protection.

NUTRITIONAL INFORMATION Calories 265, Calories from Fat 17%, Fat 5 g, Saturated Fat 1 g, Cholesterol 4 mg, Sodium 115 mg, Carbohydrates 43 g, Dietary Fiber 2 g, Total Sugars 7 g, Protein 11 g

DIABETIC EXCHANGES 2 1/2 starch, 1/2 fat-free milk, 1/2 fat

ONE STEP MACARONI AND CHEESE

Doesn't get any easier or better that my all-in-one dish comfort food recipe for Mac and Cheese.

5 cups skim milk
1 egg
1 (16-ounce) package small sea shell pasta
  or macaroni
2 1/2 cups shredded reduced-fat cheddar cheese,
  divided
Salt and pepper to taste

1 Preheat oven 350°F. Coat 2-quart baking dish with nonstick cooking spray.

2 In bowl, whisk together milk and egg.

3 In prepared dish, combine macaroni and 1 1/2 cups cheese; season to taste. Pour milk mixture over macaroni; stir well.

4 Bake, covered with foil, 45–50 minutes or until all liquid is almost absorbed. Uncover, sprinkle with remaining 1 cup cheese and bake 5 minutes more or until cheese is melted and liquid absorbed.

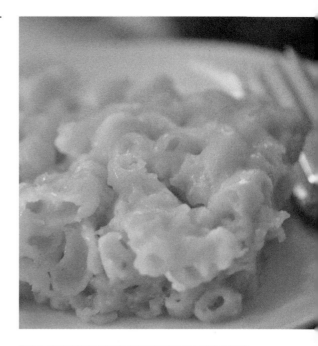

MAKES 12 (2/3 cup) servings
PREP TIME 5 minutes
COOK TIME 50 minutes

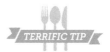
TERRIFIC TIP

If you like a touch of sweetness, add 1 tablespoon sugar. Adding a little sugar to foods helps provide a more pleasant taste, decreasing bitter or acid tastes, especially when experiencing taste changes.

· · · · · · · · · · · · · · · · ·

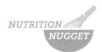
NUTRITION NUGGET

A comforting protein and carbohydrate rich dish to help fuel your day, with an added calcium boost.

NUTRITIONAL INFORMATION Calories 248, Calories from Fat 20%, Fat 5 g, Saturated Fat 3 g, Cholesterol 30 mg, Sodium 201 mg, Carbohydrates 33 g, Dietary Fiber 1 g, Total Sugars 6 g, Protein 15 g

DIABETIC EXCHANGES 2 starch, 1/2 fat-free milk, 1 lean meat

F D

SIMPLE BAKED CHICKEN

Tender chicken with gravy (tastes like chicken soup) makes a very comforting flavorsome meal. Be sure to serve with rice to soak up the last drop of gravy.

1 1/2 pounds chicken breast tenders
1/4 cup biscuit baking mix
1 tablespoon olive oil
1 teaspoon minced garlic
1 tablespoon all-purpose flour
1 (16-ounce) can low-sodium, fat-free chicken broth

1. Preheat oven 375°F. Coat 3-quart oblong baking dish with nonstick cooking spray.

2. Coat chicken in baking mix and place in prepared dish. Bake 40 minutes.

3. In small nonstick pot, combine oil and garlic; add flour. Whisk in broth, bring to boil, and cook until slightly thickened. Pour over chicken, cover with foil, and continue baking another 20–30 minutes, or until chicken is done.

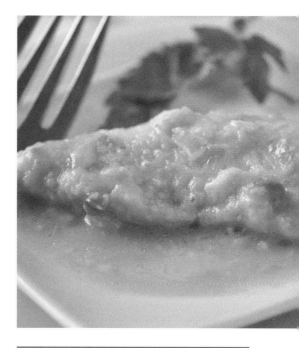

MAKES 6 servings
PREP TIME 15 minutes
COOK TIME 1 hour

TERRIFIC TIP

Add more seasoning as needed if you are experiencing taste changes.

· · · · · · · · · · · · · · · · ·

DOC'S NOTE

When not feeling well, simple, protein-rich foods such as this can help keep up your nutrition when not in the mood for anything else.

NUTRITIONAL INFORMATION Calories 173, Calories from Fat 30%, Fat 6 g, Saturated Fat 1 g, Cholesterol 73 mg, Sodium 197 mg, Carbohydrates 3 g, Dietary Fiber 0 g, Total Sugars 0 g, Protein 25 g

DIABETIC EXCHANGES 3 lean meat

F **D**

ROASTED CHICKEN AND ANGEL HAIR

The simple preparation of this one-dish roasted chicken, onion and garlic tossed with pasta recipe has the best flavor.

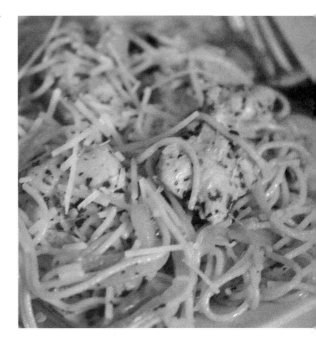

1 medium onion, thinly sliced in rings
2 teaspoons minced garlic
1 teaspoon dried basil leaves
1/4 teaspoon crushed red pepper flakes, optional
3 tablespoons olive oil, divided
1 1/2 pounds skinless, boneless chicken breasts, cut into pieces
8 ounces angel hair pasta
1/4 cup grated Parmesan cheese
Salt and pepper to taste

1 Preheat oven 400°F. Coat 2-quart oblong baking dish with nonstick cooking spray

2 In prepared dish, stir together onion, garlic, basil, red pepper and 1 tablespoon olive oil. Coat chicken with mixture. Bake chicken, uncovered, 45 minutes or until done.

3 Prepare pasta according to package directions, drain. When chicken is done, add pasta to dish with remaining olive oil, cheese, and season to taste, mixing well.

MAKES 6 (1-cup) servings
PREP TIME 15 minutes
COOK TIME 45 minutes

TERRIFIC TIP

Perk up those taste buds with red pepper flakes but may be omitted if mouth is sensitive.

· · · · · · · · · · · · · · · · ·

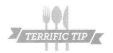
NUTRITION NUGGET

Protein rich food such as lean chicken breast is important to promote healing after chemotherapy.

NUTRITIONAL INFORMATION Calories 353, Calories from Fat 29%, Fat 11 g, Saturated Fat 2 g, Cholesterol 76 mg, Sodium 187 mg, Carbohydrates 31 g, Dietary Fiber 1 g, Total Sugars 3 g, Protein 30 g
DIABETIC EXCHANGES 2 starch, 3 lean meat

F D

CHICKEN AND DUMPLINGS

Ready in no time at all, this ultimate comfort food and soothing soup is made with rotisserie chicken and drop dumplings.

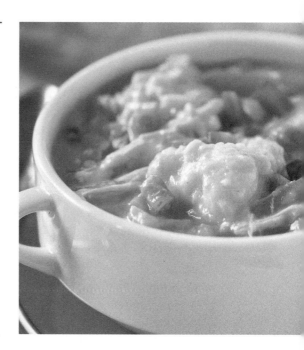

1 onion, chopped
1 cup baby carrots
1/2 teaspoon minced garlic
3 tablespoons all-purpose flour
6 cups low-sodium fat-free chicken broth, divided
1/2 teaspoon dried thyme leaves
2 cups chopped skinless rotisserie chicken breast
2 cups biscuit baking mix
2/3 cup skim milk
Salt and pepper to taste

1 In large nonstick pot coated with nonstick cooking spray, sauté onion, carrots, and garlic over medium heat until tender, about 5 minutes.

2 In small cup, stir flour and 1/3 cup broth, mixing until smooth. Gradually add flour mixture and remaining broth to pot; bring to boil. Add thyme and chicken.

3 In bowl, stir together biscuit baking mix and milk. Drop mixture by spoonfuls into boiling broth.

4 Return to boil, reduce heat, and cook, covered, carefully stirring occasionally, 15–20 minutes or until dumplings are done. Season to taste. If soup is too thick, add more chicken broth.

MAKES 8 (1-cup) servings
PREP TIME 15 minutes
COOK TIME 30 minutes

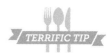
TERRIFIC TIP

A short-cut for dumplings: cut flaky biscuits into fourths and drop into boiling broth or you can even use flour tortillas cut into fourths. You can slice carrots— but I find baby carrots a time-saver.

. . . .

DOC'S NOTE

If weight loss is a problem, add fortified dry milk to add calories and protein.

NUTRITIONAL INFORMATION Calories 212, Calories from Fat 22%, Fat 5 g, Saturated Fat 1 g, Cholesterol 32 mg, Sodium 553 mg, Carbohydrates 26 g, Dietary Fiber 2 g, Total Sugars 4 g, Protein 15 g
DIABETIC EXCHANGES 1 1/2 starch, 1 vegetable, 1 1/2 lean meat

ROASTED BUTTERNUT SQUASH WITH PASTA

When you're looking for a light, simple dish, roasted butternut squash with pasta, basil and spinach is a vegetarian delight.

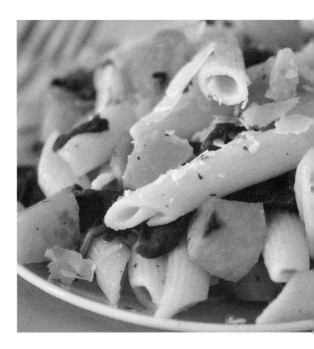

6 cups peeled, seeded, 3/4-inch cubed
  butternut squash
1 onion, coarsely chopped
Salt and pepper to taste
1 (16-ounce) package penne pasta
1 tablespoon olive oil
4 cups chopped baby spinach
1/2 cup packed fresh basil leaves, coarsely chopped
1/3 cup grated Parmesan cheese

1 Preheat oven 425°F. Line baking pan with foil and coat with nonstick cooking spray.

2 Spread squash and onion on prepared pan. Season to taste and coat squash with nonstick cooking spray. Bake 35–40 minutes until tender and lightly browned. Remove from oven; set aside.

3 Meanwhile, cook pasta according to package directions. Drain, but reserve 1 1/2 cups pasta water. Return pasta to pot and add oil, squash, onion, spinach, basil and pasta water to hot pasta. Toss well, and season to taste. Sprinkle with Parmesan cheese.

MAKES 8 (1-cup) servings
PREP TIME 15 minutes
COOK TIME 45 minutes

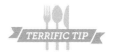

Look for pre-cut butternut squash for the ultimate short cut. Chicken broth may be used for the pasta water. Substitute 1 tablespoon dried basil for fresh, if desired.

· · · · · · · · · · · · · · · · ·

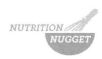

Butternut squash is rich in the antioxidant beta-carotene by its golden yellow hue.

NUTRITIONAL INFORMATION Calories 297, Calories from Fat 11%, Fat 4 g, Saturated Fat 1 g, Cholesterol 3 mg, Sodium 73 mg, Carbohydrates 57 g, Dietary Fiber 4 g, Total Sugars 5 g, Protein 10 g

DIABETIC EXCHANGES 4 starch

SWEET POTATO BISCUITS

By using baking mix, this no-fuss biscuit will be an easy breakfast or snack favorite. Best of all, the dough is incredibly easy to work with and may be pressed out with your hands.

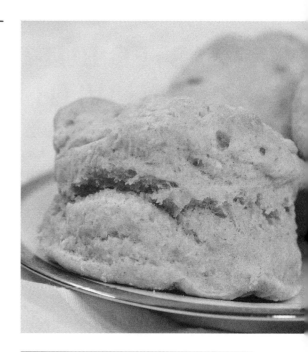

4 cups all-purpose baking mix
1/2 teaspoon ground cinnamon
1 (15-ounce) can sweet potatoes, drained, reserve 1/2 cup juice
1/2 cup skim milk

1 Preheat oven 450°F.

2 In large bowl, combine baking mix and cinnamon. Mash sweet potatoes, add to dry mixture with milk and reserved juice, mixing well.

3 Roll on floured surface until 1-inch thick. Cut with 2-inch cutter or glass, place on baking pan. Bake 10–12 minutes or until golden.

MAKES 18 biscuits
PREP TIME 10 minutes
COOK TIME 15 minutes

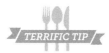
TERRIFIC TIP

Leftover cooked sweet potatoes may be used for canned. One (15-ounce) can yams equals 1 cup mashed sweet potatoes. These biscuits also make great biscuit sandwiches.

. . . .

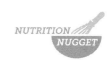
NUTRITION NUGGET

Keep these easy-to-eat biscuits in the freezer to pop out for a nutritional energy boost when feeling too tired to cook.

NUTRITIONAL INFORMATION Calories 129, Calories from Fat 27%, Fat 4 g, Saturated Fat 1 g, Cholesterol 0 mg, Sodium 343 mg, Carbohydrates 21 g, Dietary Fiber 1 g, Total Sugars 4 g, Protein 2 g
DIABETIC EXCHANGES 1 1/2 starch, 1/2 fat

LEMON ANGEL FOOD CAKE

Light, lemon and luscious, this quick-to-make cake is great to keep in the refrigerator for a snack. You can serve with fruit, if desired.

1 (6-serving) package vanilla pudding and pie filling mix
1 (8-ounce) container nonfat lemon yogurt
1 (8-ounce) container fat-free frozen whipped topping, thawed
1 (16-ounce) angel food cake (commercially bought)

1 In large bowl, whisk together pudding mix with lemon yogurt. Fold in whipped topping.

2 Slice cake horizontally into three layers. Place bottom layer on serving plate and top with one-third of lemon yogurt mixture. Repeat layers twice. Refrigerate.

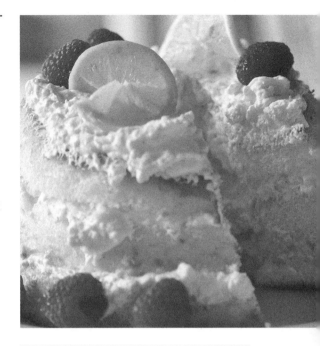

MAKES 12 servings
PREP TIME 15 minutes

TERRIFIC TIP

Use sugar free pudding and angel food cake to make the recipe diabetic-friendly.

DOC'S NOTE

Lemon and citrus flavors help reduce bitter tastes which are a common side effect of chemotherapy.

NUTRITIONAL INFORMATION Calories 210, Calories from Fat 0%, Fat 0 g, Saturated Fat 0 g, Cholesterol 0 mg, Sodium 221 mg, Carbohydrates 47 g, Dietary Fiber 0 g, Total Sugars 33 g, Protein 3 g
DIABETIC EXCHANGES 3 other carbohydrate

NEUTROPENIA

A neutropenic diet is for a weakened immune system.
No raw foods—all of these recipes include cooked meats,
seafood, fruits and vegetables to lower the risk for infection.

. . . .

What is neutropenia and how long does it last?

Do I have to go into isolation?

Is it okay to eat raw fruits and vegetables once neutropenia has subsided?

. . . .

Neutropenia, or low white blood cell count, is a common complication following a large number of treatments. Most chemotherapeutic drugs will lower your blood counts to some degree. This is because chemotherapy will destroy good cells such as white blood cells, red blood cells and platelets that are produced in the bone marrow. The goal with chemotherapy is to destroy cancer cells and allow good cells to regenerate and flourish. Unfortunately, both good and bad cells are destroyed after each treatment of chemotherapy. The nausea and vomiting is partially secondary to the destruction of cells lining the gastrointestinal tract. Hair loss is secondary to the destruction of hair follicles.

Neutropenia usually lasts four to seven days. This can vary from person to person and treatment to treatment, and it can be longer with certain leukemia treatments. Normally, it is recommended to avoid crowds and anyone that is ill until your blood counts are normal. Raw fruits, vegetables, meat, and seafood are harbingers of bacteria which, if ingested during the times your white blood cells are low, can lead to a systemic infection and should also be avoided. You can become neutropenic following successive treatments. Once your counts have recovered you can resume your normal activities and diet.

Again, during the period of neutropenia, avoid raw fruits, raw vegetables, raw meat and raw seafood, **BUT REMEMBER, YOU CAN RESUME THESE RAW FOODS AND VEGETABLES AS SOON AS YOUR COUNTS ARE UP**. I hope the recipes that follow will give you directions on what to eat during the time your white blood cell count is down and you are more susceptible to infections.

FOODS TO AVOID

- ALL RAW FOOD
- Fresh, frozen, or dried fruit
- Honey—use molasses
- Uncooked herbs and spices, including garnishes
- Raw nuts (baked products with nuts are acceptable)
- Yogurt and yogurt products with live and active cultures

ACCEPTABLE FOODS

- Processed cheese
- Canned or cooked fruits and vegetables
- All cooked or baked goods, jello, syrup, ice cream and sherbet made from pasteurized products
- Cooked hot soups
- All breads, rolls, crackers in wrappers

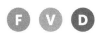

YAMCAKES

Start the morning off right with this bundle of flavor. Pancakes, sugar, spice, and everything nice—feel free to forget the syrup!

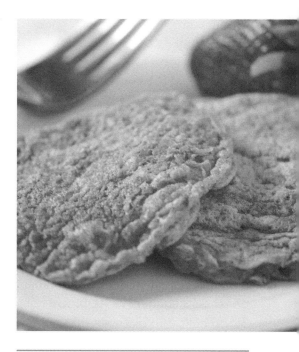

2 cups all-purpose baking mix
2 teaspoons ground cinnamon
1/2 cup mashed, canned sweet potatoes (drained)
1 (12-ounce) can evaporated skimmed milk
1 egg
1 egg white
1 tablespoon canola oil
1 teaspoon vanilla extract

1 In bowl, mix all ingredients just until combined. (The batter will be lumpy).

2 Heat large nonstick skillet or griddle coated with nonstick cooking spray. Spoon 1/4 cup batter onto pan for each pancake. Cook pancakes 1–2 minutes on each side, or until lightly browned.

MAKES 16 pancakes
PREP TIME 5 minutes
COOK TIME 5–10 minutes

TERRIFIC TIP

Make a batch of pancakes, freeze and pop in the microwave for a quick breakfast.

· · · · · · · · · · · · · · · · ·

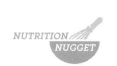

NUTRITION NUGGET

Toss in some dried fruit, pecans or chocolate chips, if desired.

NUTRITIONAL INFORMATION Calories 98, Calories from Fat 20%, Fat 2 g, Saturated Fat 0 g, Cholesterol 14 mg, Sodium 213 mg, Carbohydrates 15 g, Dietary Fiber 1 g, Total Sugars 4 g, Protein 4 g

DIABETIC EXCHANGES 1 starch

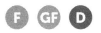

SOUTHWESTERN SOUP

This hearty soup with meat, salsa, sweet potatoes and southwestern seasonings creates a soup bursting with flavor.

1 pound ground sirloin
1 cup chopped onion
2 cups water
1 (10-ounce) can diced tomatoes and green chilies
1 cup salsa
2 cups cubed, peeled, sweet or white potatoes
1/2 teaspoon chili powder
1 teaspoon ground cumin
1/2 teaspoon minced garlic
Salt and pepper to taste
2 cups frozen corn

1. In large nonstick pot, cook meat and onion over medium heat until meat is done, about 5–7 minutes. Drain excess fat.

2. Add remaining ingredients, except corn. Bring to a boil. Reduce heat, cover, simmer about 30 minutes.

3. Add corn, continue cooking, covered, 15 minutes.

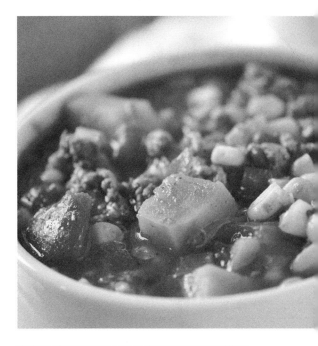

MAKES 9 (1-cup) servings
PREP TIME 10 minutes
COOK TIME 50 minutes

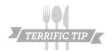

Ground turkey may be used for the ground sirloin.

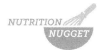

Cooked hot soups are a great way to include cooked veggies getting extra nutrients, vitamins and fiber.

NUTRITIONAL INFORMATION Calories 149, Calories from fat 17%, Fat 3 g, Saturated Fat 1 g, Cholesterol 28 mg, Sodium 289 mg, Carbohydrate 19 g, Dietary Fiber 3 g, Total Sugars 4 g, Protein 13 g

DIABETIC EXCHANGES 1 starch, 1 vegetable, 1 1/2 very lean meat

QUICK HERB CHICKEN

Select your favorite dried herbs to create this delightfully herby flavored chicken and gravy home-style dish. Serve with rice or pasta to take advantage of the gravy.

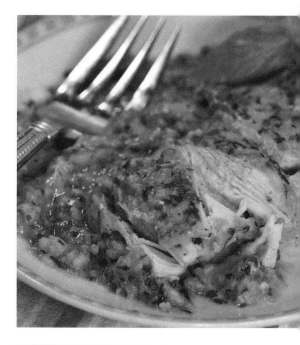

1 3/4 pounds boneless skinless chicken breasts
2 tablespoons lemon juice
1 tablespoon minced garlic
Salt and pepper to taste
1/2 cup all-purpose flour
1 tablespoon olive oil
2 cups fat-free chicken broth
1 tablespoon Dijon mustard
2-3 tablespoons dried herbs (basil, oregano, or thyme)

1 In plastic zip-top bag, combine chicken, lemon juice, garlic and season to taste. Coat seasoned chicken in flour.

2 In large nonstick skillet coated with nonstick cooking spray, heat oil and brown chicken on each side, about 5 minutes.

3 In small bowl, combine broth, mustard, and herbs; add to skillet. Bring to boil, lower heat, cover and cook until chicken is tender, 20 minutes.

MAKES 4 servings
PREP TIME 15 minutes
COOK TIME 25 minutes

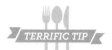

TERRIFIC TIP

Pasta tossed with olive oil makes a great side dish.

· · · · · · · · · · · · · · · · ·

DOC'S NOTE

If you are experiencing taste changes adding extra seasonings to foods may help stimulate your appetite and perk up your taste buds—avoid fresh, uncooked herbs and spices.

NUTRITIONAL INFORMATION Calories 230, Calories from Fat 24%, Fat 6 g, Saturated Fat 1 g, Cholesterol 85 mg, Sodium 298 mg, Carbohydrates 11 g, Dietary Fiber 1 g, Total Sugars 1 g, Protein 30 g
DIABETIC EXCHANGES 1 starch, 4 lean meat

F GF

PULLED CHICKEN

Forget barbecue when you can instantly whip up this awesome and simple pulled chicken recipe.

1 cup chopped onion
1/2 teaspoon minced garlic
2 tablespoons cider vinegar
1/2 cup chili sauce
1 tablespoon light brown sugar
1 teaspoon cocoa
1/2 teaspoon ground cumin
1/2 cup low-sodium fat-free chicken broth
2 cups shredded skinless rotisserie chicken breast

1 In nonstick pot coated with nonstick cooking spray, sauté onion until tender. Add remaining ingredients except chicken, stirring. Cook about 7 minutes.

2 Add chicken and continue cooking until well heated.

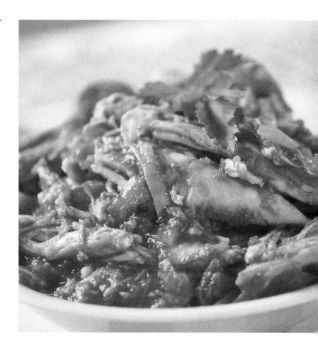

MAKES 4 (3/4-cup) servings
PREP TIME 10 minutes
COOK TIME 15 minutes

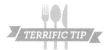

Chili sauce is found where ketchup is in the grocery. You may substitute ketchup for chili sauce. Serve on sandwiches, sliders or as an entrée.

. . . .

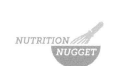

If serving as sandwiches, look for 100% whole-wheat bread and buns for bonus fiber and nutrition content.

NUTRITIONAL INFORMATION Calories 170 Calories from Fat 14% Fat 3g Saturated Fat 1g Cholesterol 63mg Sodium 821mg Carbohydrates 16g Dietary Fiber 1g Total Sugars 11g Protein 21g

DIABETIC EXCHANGES 1 other carbohydrate, 3 lean meat

QUICK CHICKEN LASAGNA

If you don't feel like cooking, try this 'so simple' 5-ingredient, throw-together lasagna, a favorite fantastic dinner.

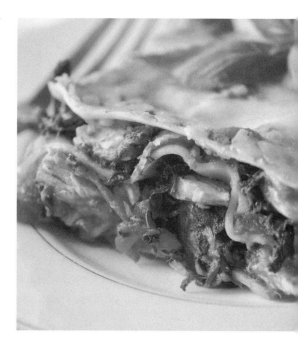

4 cups cooked cubed or shredded skinless chicken breast (rotisserie chicken)
6 cups marinara sauce
1 (8-ounce) package no-boil lasagna noodles
1 3/4 cups shredded part-skim mozzarella cheese
2 (10-ounce) packages chopped spinach, thawed and drained

1 Preheat oven 350°F. Coat oblong baking dish with nonstick cooking spray.

2 In large bowl, combine chicken and marinara sauce.

3 In prepared dish, spread thin layer of sauce. Top with layer of noodles, more chicken sauce, mozzarella cheese, and half the spinach.

4 Repeat layering with noodles, chicken sauce, cheese, and remaining spinach. Continue with remaining noodles, sauce, and cheese.

5 Bake, covered, 50 minutes. Uncover and bake 5 minutes or until bubbly.

MAKES 10 servings
PREP TIME 15 minutes
COOK TIME 1 hour

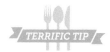

The perfect make-ahead 'TV dinner' meal. To freeze: Cool to room temperature, cut in individual portions, wrap, label and freeze.

. . . .

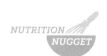

By using "healthy" marinara sauce you will help to lower your sodium and sugar intake.

NUTRITIONAL INFORMATION Calories 268, Calories from Fat 48%, Fat 5 g, Saturated Fat 2 g, Cholesterol 48 mg, Sodium 588 mg, Carbohydrates 31 g, Dietary Fiber 4 g, Total Sugars 9 g, Protein 24 g
DIABETIC EXCHANGES 2 starch, 3 very lean meat

CHICKEN WITH LEMON CAPER SAUCE

Think of this as a delicious smothered chicken with fancy flair. Serve with rice or over angel hair pasta tossed with olive oil and garlic.

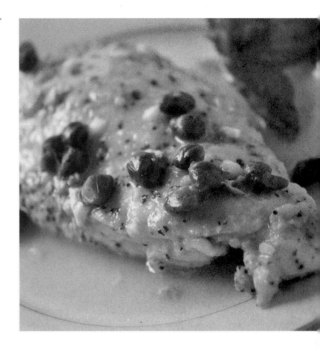

1/3 cup all-purpose flour
Salt and pepper to taste
6 (4–5-ounce) boneless, skinless chicken breasts, pounded thin, if desired
2 tablespoons olive oil
1 teaspoon minced garlic
1 1/2 cups low-sodium, fat-free chicken broth
1/2 cup lemon juice
1/2 cup wine or low-sodium, fat-free chicken broth
1/4 cup capers, drained

1 In plastic bag, combine flour and season to taste. Add chicken to coat.

2 In large nonstick skillet coated with nonstick cooking spray, heat oil, and cook chicken breasts over medium high heat, until lightly brown, about 3–4 minutes each side. Remove chicken to plate.

3 To pan, add garlic, broth, lemon juice, wine and capers. Bring to boil, scrapping pan for loose bits. Return chicken to pan, reduce heat, cover, and simmer until chicken is tender, about 10–15 minutes.

MAKES 6 (4-ounce) servings
PREP TIME 10 minutes
COOK TIME 20 minutes

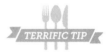

Look for thin chicken breasts in the store. To pound chicken, use meat pounder or something hard, cover chicken with wax paper and pound to flatten—this tenderizes chicken.

DOC'S NOTE

This protein rich meal helps to ensure growth, to repair body tissue, and to maintain a healthy immune system.

NUTRITIONAL INFORMATION Calories 209, Calories from Fat 34%, Fat 8 g, Saturated Fat 1 g, Cholesterol 73 mg, Sodium 222 mg, Carbohydrates 7 g, Dietary Fiber 0 g, Total Sugars 1 g, Protein 25 g

DIABETIC EXCHANGES 1/2 starch, 3 lean meat

ROASTED SEASONED SALMON

This easy-to-make recipe with simple seasonings perk up salmon with a sweet and spicy rub.

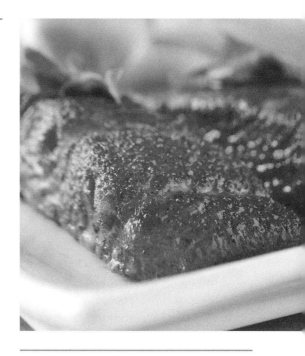

2 tablespoons light brown sugar
4 teaspoons chili powder
1 teaspoon ground cumin
1/4 teaspoon ground cinnamon
Salt and pepper to taste
4 (6-ounce) salmon fillets

1 Preheat oven 400°F. Coat an 11×7×2-inch baking dish with nonstick cooking spray.

2 In small bowl, mix together brown sugar, chili powder, cumin, cinnamon and season to taste. Rub over salmon and place in prepared dish.

3 Bake 12–15 minutes or until fish flakes easily when tested with fork.

MAKES 4 servings
PREP TIME 5 minutes
COOK TIME 15 minutes

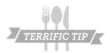

Make sure your salmon, as with all meat and seafood, is thoroughly cooked to kill all bacteria.

. . . .

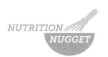

At least two servings of fish (fatty fish preferred) per week for heart health is the recommended intake by the American Heart Association.

NUTRITIONAL INFORMATION Calories 257, Calories from Fat 29%, Fat 8 g, Saturated Fat 1 g, Cholesterol 80 mg, Sodium 177 mg, Carbohydrates 8 g, Dietary Fiber 1 g, Total Sugars 7 g, Protein 36 g

DIABETIC EXCHANGES 2 vegetable, 1 fat

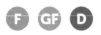

SPICY BAKED FISH

A quick and easy delicious method to prepare your favorite fish.

1 pound fish fillets
2 tablespoons light mayonnaise
1 teaspoon lemon juice
1/2 teaspoon Dijon mustard
1/2 teaspoon garlic powder
1/8 teaspoon cayenne pepper
Dash Worcestershire sauce
Paprika, to sprinkle

1 Preheat oven 500°F. Line baking pan with foil and coat with nonstick cooking spray.

2 Rinse fish fillets, and pat dry. In small dish, combine mayonnaise, lemon juice, mustard, garlic powder, cayenne and Worcestershire sauce.

3 Lay fish in prepared pan. Spread mayonnaise mixture evenly over fish. If time permitted let sit 30 minutes. Sprinkle with paprika.

4 Bake 10-15 minutes, or until fish flakes easily with a fork. Serve immediately.

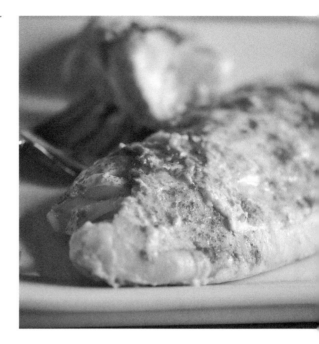

MAKES 4 servings
PREP TIME 10 minutes
COOK TIME 15 minutes

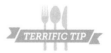

TERRIFIC TIP

Don't overcook fish—cook it just until it begins to flake. Fish suggesetions include trout, catfish or any mild-flavored fish.

. . . .

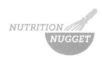

NUTRITION NUGGET

Fish options high in heart-healthy omega-3 fatty acids include mackerel and rainbow trout.

NUTRITIONAL INFORMATION Calories 108, Calories from Fat 29%, Fat 3 g, Saturated Fat 0 g, Cholesterol 25 mg, Sodium 142 mg, Carbohydrates 2 g, Dietary Fiber 0 g, Total Sugars 0 g, Protein 17 g

DIABETIC EXCHANGES 3 very lean meat

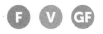

MAKES 5 servings

PREP TIME 5 minutes | **COOK TIME** 10 minutes

BAKED PEACH DELIGHT

A great substitute for fresh fruit—adjust recipe according to number of peach halves in the can. Can serve with nonfat frozen yogurt.

>   1 (16-ounce) can peach halves, drained (5 halves)
>   5 tablespoons peanut butter
>   5 teaspoons light brown sugar

1 Preheat oven 350°F.

2 Place peach halves in baking dish, pit-side up. Spread 1 tablespoon peanut butter on each peach half and sprinkle each with 1 teaspoon brown sugar. Bake until peanut butter and brown sugar melt, about 5–10 minutes.

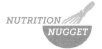

NUTRITION NUGGET

The yellow-orange color of peaches indicates they are rich in beta-carotene, protecting the body against free radicals. Remember you can resume eating raw foods and vegetables once your counts are up.

NUTRITIONAL INFORMATION Calories 142, Calories from Fat 47%, Fat 8 g, Saturated Fat 2 g, Cholesterol 0 mg, Sodium 74 mg, Carbohydrates 16 g, Dietary Fiber 2 g, Total Sugars 13 g, Protein 4 g

DIABETIC EXCHANGES 1 fruit, 1/2 lean meat, 1 fat

MAKES 5 servings

PREP TIME 2 minutes | **COOK TIME** 2 minutes

HOT COCOA DRINK SUPPLEMENT

Packages of cocoa mix turn these drinks into chocolate delights. A great drink on those cold winter mornings that will give you extra calories, vitamins, and minerals. Check my tip below for more drink options.

>   1 (8-ounce) can nutritional energy drink supplement
>   1 package hot cocoa mix

1 Pour drink supplement in large microwaveable mug, and microwave until very hot.

2 Gradually stir in the cocoa mix until well blended. Let cool to room temperature if needed.

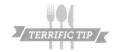

TERRIFIC TIP

For coffee lovers, stir 1/2 teaspoon instant coffee to hot chocolate.
***For Cocoa Smoothie:** add cocoa mix to 1/2 cup chilled chocolate nutritional energy drink supplement with 1/2 cup ice cubes and blend in blender until smooth.*

NUTRITIONAL INFORMATION Calories 333, Calories from Fat 15%, Fat 6 g, Saturated Fat 2 g, Cholesterol 4 mg, Sodium 275 mg, Carbohydrates 59 g, Dietary Fiber 1 g, Total Sugars 40 g, Protein 10 g

DIABETIC EXCHANGES 4 other carbohydrate

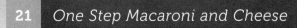

NAUSEA

Easier to digest recipes that are mild, low fiber foods with little odor and light in flavor to help decrease nausea, vomiting and diarrhea.

. . . .

Will it ever stop?

Should I stop eating and drinking altogether?

What should I eat and drink?

Is it alright to take Immodium, Lomotil or Pepto Bismol?

My rectum is sore, what can I do?

. . . .

Diarrhea can follow certain chemotherapy or radiation treatments. This can be a problem with certain drugs such as 5-FU, CPT-11 and antibiotics. If the diarrhea starts, the first thing to do is to stop all intake of high fiber foods—such as nuts, seeds, whole grains, legumes, dried fruit and raw fruits and vegetables—stool softeners or laxatives. Follow your doctors' instructions with regards to Lomotil, Immodium, or Pepto Bismol. Start clear liquids after fasting two to four hours. Force fluids up to eight to ten glasses per day. Water, clear soup, broth, flat soda or a sports drink are excellent fluids to replace those lost by diarrhea. Avoid dairy products since they tend to make diarrhea worse. Avoid gassy foods and carbonated beverages. Hot and cold beverages, alcohol, coffee and cigarettes tend to aggravate diarrhea. Be sure to sip fluids throughout the day to prevent dehydration.

Bananas, rice, applesauce and toast (known as the B.R.A.T. diet) are good foods to begin eating following a decrease in your diarrhea. Once you are tolerating these foods, progress to bland low fiber foods, such as chicken without the skin, scrambled eggs, and canned or cooked fruits without skins. Crackers, pasta without sauce, white bread or gelatins are good choices. Try to avoid foods high in fiber, such as grains, raw vegetables, whole-wheat, raw fruit, oatmeal and brown rice.

Once your diarrhea has subsided, you can adjust your diet accordingly. Foods low in fiber and fat are helpful in decreasing your diarrhea. If your rectum becomes red or sore, use a commercial wet towel without alcohol and avoid dry toilet paper. Desitin or a combination of Aquaphor and Questran in a 9 to 1 ratio, will act as a protective barrier to your perirectal area. Ask your physician to prescribe these medications.

If your diarrhea continues without relief for greater than twenty-four hours, please notify your physician. Here are some recipes and suggestions that follow to help get you regulated and eating healthy again.

POINTS TO REMEMBER

- Eat chicken soup or bouillon cubes dissolved in water.
- Eat bland, high-protein foods.
- Eat smaller mini meals throughout the day to see what you can tolerate.
- Eat high-calorie, low-fiber foods.

- Avoid citrus juices and carbonated beverages. An alternative to carbonated drinks is mineral water with a splash of fruit juices, which is both bubbly and tasty.

- Avoid raw vegetables and fruits, and high fiber foods, nuts, onions, garlic, and gaseous vegetables.

- Avoid spicy foods.

- Avoid greasy, fatty, or fried foods.

- Drink beverages frequently, in small amounts, and at room temperature.

- Limit caffeine intake.

- Choose low fiber light foods like fish, chicken, eggs, bananas, potatoes, low fiber cereals, crackers, refined bread and flour products. Crackers with peanut butter or cheese sometimes works.

- Do minimal activity after meals.

- Ginger can be soothing to the stomach: gingersnaps, ginger candy.

- Drink plenty of mild, clear, non-carbonated liquids throughout the day. Drink liquids at room temperature, as they are better tolerated than hot or cold beverages. Flat soda is another good choice.

- Limit milk.

- Avoid drinks and foods that cause gas, such as carbonated drinks, chewing gum and gas-forming vegetables (broccoli, cauliflower, cabbage, Brussels sprouts and beans). Drink carbonated beverages if you leave them open for at least 10 minutes before drinking.

- Drink and eat high-sodium foods such as broths, soups, sports drinks, crackers, baked chips and pretzels.

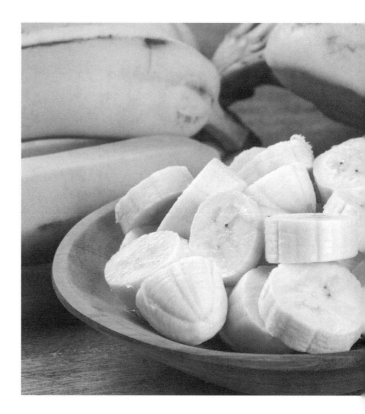

- Drink and eat high-potassium foods such as fruit juices and nectars, sports drinks, potatoes without the skin, and bananas.

- Eat foods high in pectin such as applesauce and bananas.

- Avoid chewing gums, sugar-free gums, and all candies made with sorbitol.

- Be sure to sip fluids throughout the day to prevent dehydration.

- When recommended by a healthcare practitioner, soluble fiber can be used to relieve mild to moderate diarrhea. Soluble fiber soaks up a significant amount of water in the digestive tract causing stool to be more firm and pass slower. Soluble fiber sources include: Legumes, oats, bananas, apples, berries, broccoli, carrots, potatoes and yams (without skins).

SOME FOODS TO INCLUDE

- Toast, crackers or pretzels
- Flavored gelatin
- Applesauce
- Skinless chicken
- Clear liquids
- Bananas
- Rice
- Plums, peaches, watermelon, cantaloupe

WHEN YOU ARE FEELING QUEASY

If you experience nausea and vomiting, try to drink fluids to prevent dehydration. Sip water, juices, and other clear, calorie-containing liquids throughout the day. You may tolerate clear, cool liquids better than very hot or icy fluids. When you have stopped vomiting, try eating easy to digest foods such as clear liquids, crackers, gelatin, and plain toast.

POINTS TO REMEMBER

- Eat six to eight small meals a day, instead of three large meals.
- Eat dry foods, such as crackers, toast, dry cereals, pretzels or bread sticks, when you wake up and every few hours during the day.
- Eat foods that do not have a strong odor.
- Eat cool foods instead of hot spicy foods.
- Avoid foods that are overly sweet, greasy, fried, or spicy, such as rich desserts and French fries.
- Sit up or recline with your head raised for at least 1 hour after eating if you need to rest.

- Sip clear liquids frequently to prevent dehydration.
- Ask your doctor about medications that prevent or stop nausea.
- Try bland, soft, easy-to-digest foods on scheduled treatment days. Foods such as cream of wheat and chicken noodle soup with saltine crackers may be better tolerated than heavy meals.
- Avoid eating in a room that is warm, or that has cooking odors or other smells. Cook outside on the grill or use boiling bags to reduce cooking odors.
- Rinse your mouth before and after meals.
- Suck on hard candy, such as peppermint or lemon, if there is a bad taste in your mouth.
- Drink eight or more cups of liquid each day if you can. Drink an additional half cup to one cup of liquid for each episode of vomiting. Try sipping liquids 30 to 60 minutes after eating solid food.
- Ginger is an herb recognized to help with nausea. Try drinking ginger tea or flat ginger ale.

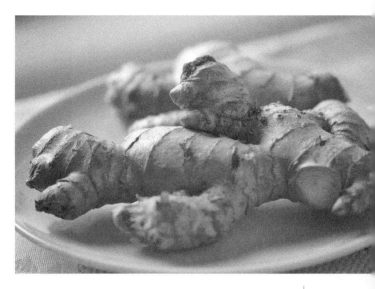

FIGHT NAUSEA WITH THESE INGREDIENTS:

Apple: Fiber helps your body clear out chemicals that could be causing your nausea. However, too much fiber can make nausea worse. Gala apples and other crunchy fruits and vegetables are good fiber-rich foods to snack on. Applesauce or apple juice may be appropriate if solid foods are hard to digest.

Bananas: Rich in potassium, bananas contain this needed nutrient when you are nauseous and especially when dehydrated from vomiting and diarrhea. Bananas are often the recommended food to start with once ready to eat solid foods from a clear or liquid diet.

Chicken Broth: Chicken soup may be too heavy on your stomach when feeling nauseous, so give low fat chicken broth a try. Chicken bouillon is another good option as it is quick to prepare, easy to keep on hand, and less likely to go bad.

Chilled Foods: Chilled or room temperature foods such as sandwiches, salads, sorbet, and popsicles tend to be much better tolerated than warm or hot foods when feeling nauseous.

Crackers: Starchy foods like crackers and toast help settle nausea by absorbing stomach acids. Keep a stash of saltine crackers on the go and on your bedside table to combat morning nausea.

Ginger: Ginger is an herb recognized to help with nausea and sooth the stomach. Try drinking ginger tea, flat ginger ale, gingersnap cookies, ginger candy, or pickled ginger.

Lemon: The tart taste or even smell of lemon can be helpful to alleviate nausea. Sniff cut up lemon slices or sip on lemon water or tea, even sucking on sour lemon candies may help.

Nuts: Nuts are packed with easy to digest protein, which your body needs to stave off nausea. Peanut butter is also a quick protein and energy source when yours is low.

Peppermint: Though the research findings are slim, many people agree that peppermint flavored food and drinks such as candy or mint tea help calm a nauseous stomach.

Sports Drinks: Sports drinks help replenish the electrolytes sodium and potassium that your body needs when nauseous and vomiting.

Water: Stay hydrated with plain water to combat headache-induced nausea. Keep your sips small until your stomach can handle larger amounts.

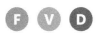

GINGERBREAD MUFFINS

This awesome muffin has all the flavor of your favorite spiced cookie in a moist anytime snack or breakfast muffin.

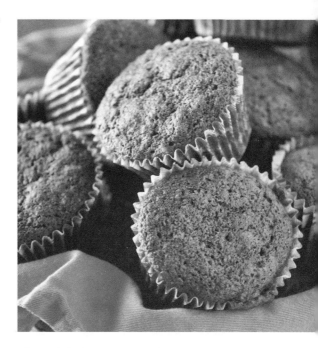

1 1/2 cups whole-wheat flour
1 cup all-purpose flour
1 teaspoon ground ginger
1 teaspoon ground cinnamon
1/2 teaspoon ground cloves, optional
1/2 cup sugar
1/3 cup canola oil
1 cup light molasses
2 eggs
1 cup boiling water
2 teaspoons baking soda

1 Preheat oven 325°F. Coat muffin pans with nonstick cooking spray or line with papers.

2 In large bowl, combine both flours, ginger, cinnamon, and cloves, if desired. Set aside.

3 In medium bowl, whisk together sugar and oil. Add molasses and eggs whisking until blended. In glass measuring cup combine water and baking soda. Stir to dissolve. Pour in egg mixture and whisk until blended. Add egg mixture to flour mixture, stirring just until combined.

4 Spoon batter into paper lined tins, filling 1/2–3/4 full. Bake 20–25 minutes or until inserted toothpick comes out clean.

MAKES 20 muffins
PREP TIME 15 minutes
COOK TIME 25 minutes

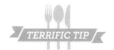

Freeze muffins to pop out when not feeling well and need a boost. All-purpose flour may be used, if that's what you have.

DOC'S NOTE

Ginger has been shown to help nausea symptoms so these muffins may be just the ticket to feeling better.

NUTRITIONAL INFORMATION Calories 161, Calories from Fat 25%, Fat 5 g, Saturated Fat 0 g, Cholesterol 19 mg, Sodium 140 mg, Carbohydrates 28 g, Dietary Fiber 1 g, Total Sugars 14 g, Protein 2 g

DIABETIC EXCHANGES 2 starch, 1/2 fat

EASY BANANA BREAD

Biscuit baking mix keeps this exceptional quick bread recipe simple, cream cheese gives it a rich flavor and ripe bananas make it moist.

4 ounces reduced-fat cream cheese
3/4 cup light brown sugar
2 eggs
1 1/2 cups mashed bananas
1 3/4 cups biscuit baking mix
1 teaspoon ground cinnamon
1 cup chopped pecans or walnuts, optional

1 Preheat oven 350°F. Coat 9×5×3-inch loaf pan with nonstick cooking spray.

2 In large mixing bowl, mix together cream cheese and brown sugar until light and fluffy. Beat in eggs and bananas. Stir in biscuit mix, cinnamon and nuts, if using, until just blended. Transfer to prepared pan.

3 Bake 40–45 minutes or until toothpick inserted in center comes out clean.

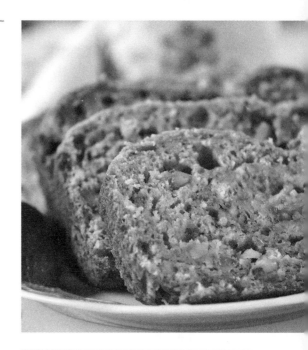

MAKES 16 slices
PREP TIME 10 minutes
COOK TIME 45 minutes

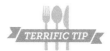

Have over-ripe bananas? Freeze to pull out to make banana bread at any time. Freeze with or without peeling in plastic freezer zip-top bags.

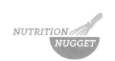

Bananas are a great source of potassium. They are easily digested by virtually everyone.

NUTRITIONAL INFORMATION Calories 138, Calories from Fat 25%, Fat 4 g, Saturated Fat 2 g, Cholesterol 28 mg, Sodium 205 mg, Carbohydrates 24 g, Dietary Fiber 1 g, Total Sugars 13 g, Protein 3 g
DIABETIC EXCHANGES 1 starch, 1/2 fruit, 1/2 fat

BANANA PANCAKES

A light pancake hits the spot when you aren't feeling great. If desired, top with sliced bananas.

1 cup all-purpose flour
1/2 cup whole-wheat flour
2 teaspoons baking powder
1/2 teaspoon baking soda
2 ripe bananas, mashed
1 1/4 cups buttermilk
1 egg
1 tablespoon canola oil
1 tablespoon brown sugar

1. In large bowl, whisk together flours, baking powder, and baking soda.

2. In another bowl, whisk together mashed bananas, buttermilk, egg, oil, and brown sugar. Pour into dry ingredients and mix until just combined, do not over mix.

3. Heat skillet or griddle over medium heat with nonstick cooking spray. Pour 1/4 cup batter into skillet to form pancakes. Cook until bubbles. Flip and cook other side until golden brown.

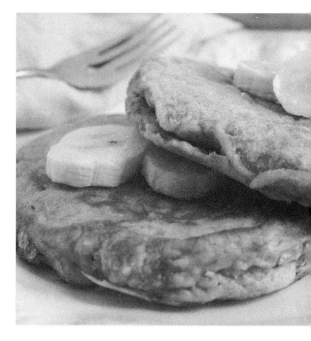

MAKES 10 (1-pancake) servings
PREP TIME 10 minutes
COOK TIME 10 minutes

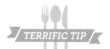
TERRIFIC TIP

Have extra pancakes? They freeze well so you can pop out for an easy breakfast or snack. If you don't have buttermilk, add 1 tablespoon lemon juice to 1 cup skim milk.

. . . .

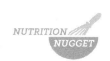
NUTRITION **NUGGET**

Trying using whole-wheat flour or half of each flour, as tolerated, to boost nutrition.

NUTRITIONAL INFORMATION Calories 124, Calories from Fat 18%, Fat 2 g, Saturated Fat 0 g, Cholesterol 20 mg, Sodium 183 mg, Carbohydrates 22 g, Dietary Fiber 2 g, Total Sugars 6 g, Protein 4 g

DIABETIC EXCHANGES 1 1/2 starch

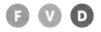

F **V** **D**	MAKES **8 servings**
F **V**	MAKES **1 egg in the bread**

PREP TIME **15 minutes** | COOK TIME **25 minutes**

PREP TIME **5 minutes** | COOK TIME **5 minutes**

BAKED FRENCH TOAST

Not feeling well but want breakfast waiting for you in the morning? Whip up this delicious dish the night before and pop in the oven the next day. The orange juice and maple syrup make this a light, not-too-sweet dish.

> 3 tablespoons butter, melted
> 1/3 cup maple syrup
> 1 teaspoon ground cinnamon
> 1 egg
> 4 egg whites
> 1 cup orange juice
> 8 slices bread

1 Preheat oven 375°F. In 13×9×2-inch baking pan, combine butter and syrup; sprinkle with cinnamon.

2 In large bowl, whisk together egg, egg whites, and orange juice. Dip bread into egg mixture and arrange in single layer in prepared pan. Bake 20–25 minutes, or until bread is light brown.

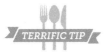

If your mouth is sore, orange juice might irritate your mouth so try using skim milk to replace juice.

NUTRITIONAL INFORMATION Calories 185, Calories from Fat 29%, Fat 6 g, Saturated Fat 1 g, Cholesterol 27 mg, Sodium 248 mg, Carbohydrates 28 g, Dietary Fiber 1 g, Total Sugars 1 g, Protein 5 g

DIABETIC EXCHANGES 1 starch, 1/2 fruit, 1/2 other carbohydrate, 1 fat

EGG IN THE BREAD

Sometimes a simple egg and bread is easy-to-eat and satisfying.

> 1 slice white or whole-wheat bread
> 1 teaspoon butter
> 1 egg
> Salt and pepper to taste

1 Cut 2-inch hole in center of bread.

2 In small nonstick pan coated with nonstick cooking spray, heat butter until melted and sizzling. Place bread in pan and break egg into the hole. Place cut out portion of bread in pan, and cook also.

3 Cook over medium heat until egg white is set, about 3 minutes. Turn over with spatula, and cook on the other side until egg is done and set. Season to taste.

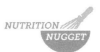

NUTRITION NUGGET

The simple egg is actually the perfect protein— containing every essential amino acid in the right ratio.

NUTRITIONAL INFORMATION Calories 172, Calories from Fat 50%, Fat 9 g, Saturated Fat 4 g, Cholesterol 196 mg, Sodium 228 mg, Carbohydrates 13 g, Dietary Fiber 1 g, Total Sugars 1 g, Protein 9 g

DIABETIC EXCHANGES 1 starch, 1 lean meat, 1 fat

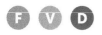

SCRAMBLED EGG MUFFIN

A quick breakfast that is a little more than scrambled eggs but still easily tolerated. You can add Canadian bacon and other ingredients as you feel better.

1 egg
1 egg white
Salt and pepper to taste
1 English muffin half (try whole-wheat)
1 tablespoon reduced-fat shredded Cheddar cheese

1 Preheat oven 350°F.

2 In small bowl, whisk together egg and egg white. In nonstick skillet coated with nonstick cooking spray, scramble eggs until done. Season to taste.

3 Carefully spoon egg mixture onto top of muffin half. Sprinkle with cheese.

4 Place muffin on nonstick baking sheet. Bake 5 minutes or until heated and cheese melted.

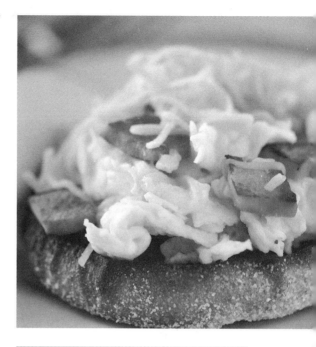

MAKES 1 egg muffin
PREP TIME 5 minutes
COOK TIME 10 minutes

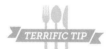

To freeze for another quick meal: Before baking, wrap individually, and freeze. Don't limit to only breakfast as light meals are great all day long.

· · · · · · · · · · · · · · · ·

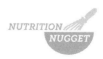

Add slice of chicken or turkey or Canadian bacon if feeling better, for added protein.

NUTRITIONAL INFORMATION Calories 170, Calories from Fat 37%, Fat 7 g, Saturated Fat 2 g, Cholesterol 213 mg, Sodium 300 mg, Carbohydrates 13 g, Dietary Fiber 1 g, Total Sugars 1 g, Protein 14 g

DIABETIC EXCHANGES 1 carbohydrate, 2 lean meat

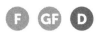

ROASTED CHICKEN SOUP WITH RICE

With rotisserie chicken and canned broth, you can easily make this nourishing and comforting chicken soup.

1 cup chopped onion
1 cup chopped carrots
1 cup chopped celery
6 cups low-sodium, fat-free chicken broth
1/4 teaspoon dried thyme leaves
1/4 cup rice
2 cups diced skinless rotisserie chicken breast
Salt and pepper to taste

1. In large nonstick pot coated with nonstick cooking spray, sauté onion, carrots, and celery 5–7 minutes or until tender. Add broth and thyme, bring to boil and add rice.

2. Lower heat, cover and cook about 15 minutes or until rice is tender. Add chicken and heat 5 minutes. Season to taste.

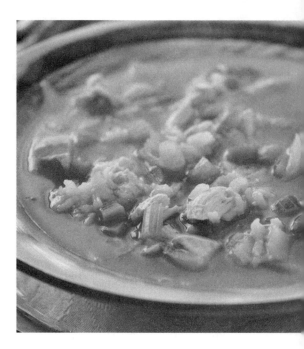

MAKES **8 (1-cup) servings**
PREP TIME **10 minutes**
COOK TIME **25 minutes**

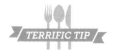

Keep bouillon cubes or jars of bouillon on hand for a plain cup of soup until feeling better.

· · · · · · · · · · · · · · · · ·

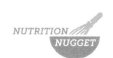

Protein rich soups and broths are excellent to replenish nutrients when experiencing diarrhea.

NUTRITIONAL INFORMATION Calories 98, Calories from Fat 14%, Fat 1 g, Saturated Fat 0 g, Cholesterol 32 mg, Sodium 189 mg, Carbohydrates 8 g, Dietary Fiber 1 g, Total Sugars 2 g, Protein 13 g

DIABETIC EXCHANGES 1/2 starch, 1 1/2 lean meat

F D

CHICKEN SCALLOPINI

Stress-free, light and flavor packed chicken when you want a more substantial, but not too rich, meal.

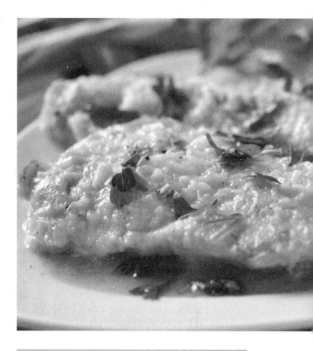

1/4 cup all-purpose flour
1/2 teaspoon garlic powder
1 1/4 pounds boneless, skinless chicken breasts, pounded thin (about four)
2 tablespoons olive oil
1 1/4 cups fat-free chicken broth
2 tablespoons lemon juice

1 In shallow bowl, combine flour, and garlic powder. Coat chicken with flour mixture.

2 In large nonstick skillet coated with nonstick cooking spray, heat oil and cook chicken breasts until lightly browned, about 4 minutes each side.

3 Add broth, bring to boil, reduce heat, cover, and simmer until chicken is tender, 15–20 minutes. Add lemon juice and heat.

MAKES **4 servings**
PREP TIME **10 minutes**
COOK TIME **30 minutes**

TERRIFIC TIP

You can buy thin chicken breasts in the grocery instead of pounding them.

DOC'S NOTE

If feeling queasy, sip water, juices, and other clear, calorie-containing liquids throughout the day.

NUTRITIONAL INFORMATION Calories 258, Calories from Fat 38%, Fat 11g, Saturated Fat 2g, Cholesterol 91mg, Sodium 287mg, Carbohydrates 7g, Dietary Fiber 1g, Total Sugars 0g, Protein 32g

DIABETIC EXCHANGES 1/2 starch, 4 lean meat

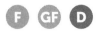

GLAZED GINGER CHICKEN

If you're feeling better, this simple infused ginger chicken might be your next step.

2 teaspoons ground ginger
4 tablespoons hoisin sauce
2 teaspoons low-sodium soy sauce
2 teaspoons olive oil
2 pounds boneless skinless chicken breast tenders (or thighs)

1 In resealable plastic bag, mix ginger, hoisin sauce, soy sauce and olive oil. Add chicken, mixing well. Marinate in refrigerator one hour or longer as time permits.

2 *To grill:* place chicken on preheated grill at low to medium. Grill each side 4-6 minutes. Remove from grill and let sit 5 minutes. If desired, broil in oven on foil lined pan.

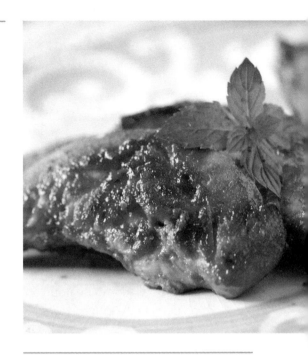

MAKES **8 servings**

PREP TIME **5 minutes + time to marinate**

COOK TIME **15 minutes**

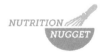

TERRIFIC TIP

Leftovers make great sandwiches, wraps or top salads.

· · · · · · · · · · · · · · · ·

NUTRITION NUGGET

Known for its anti-nausea affects, this ginger-rich chicken is also a good source of protein.

NUTRITIONAL INFORMATION Calories 152, Calories from Fat 25%, Fat 4 g, Saturated Fat 1 g, Cholesterol 73 mg, Sodium 204 mg, Carbohydrates 3 g, Dietary Fiber 0 g, Total Sugars 2 g, Protein 24 g

DIABETIC EXCHANGES 3 lean meat

OVEN FRIED CRUNCHY CHICKEN

Enjoy incredibly tasty, crunchy oven fried chicken with this hassle-free recipe.

1/2 cup nonfat plain yogurt
1 (1-ounce) packet Ranch style dressing mix
2 pounds boneless skinless chicken cutlets (or pounded thin)
3 cups corn flakes
3 tablespoons all-purpose flour
1 teaspoon paprika
Salt and pepper to taste

1 In large plastic resealable bag mix together yogurt and Ranch dressing mix. Add chicken, mixing well to cover and refrigerate 2 hours or overnight, time permitting.

2 Preheat oven 375°F. Line baking pan with foil and coat with nonstick cooking spray.

3 Crush corn flakes into crumbs and mix with flour and paprika; season to taste. Remove chicken and coat with corn flake crumb mixture. Place on prepared pan and refrigerate until ready to bake.

4 Bake 45–50 minutes or until tender and golden brown.

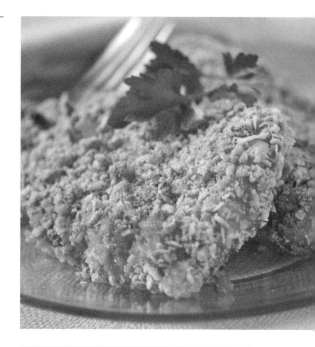

MAKES **8 servings**
PREP TIME **15 minutes + time to marinate**
COOK TIME **50 minutes**

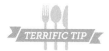
TERRIFIC TIP

If you need to rest after eating a meal, sit up or recline with your head raised for at least 1 hour to limit stomach distress.

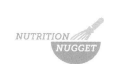
NUTRITION NUGGET

The Ranch dressing seasons the chicken with extra flavor; however, if you aren't feeling well, you can just use salt and pepper or other spices you can tolerate.

NUTRITIONAL INFORMATION Calories 193, Calories from Fat 15%, Fat 3 g, Saturated Fat 1 g, Cholesterol 73 mg, Sodium 546 mg, Carbohydrates 14 g, Dietary Fiber 0 g, Total Sugars 2 g, Protein 26 g

DIABETIC EXCHANGES 1 starch, 3 lean meat

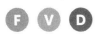

RICE NOODLE MEDLEY

You'll thoroughly enjoy this combination of rice and noodles with a toasty flavor.

1 cup uncooked rice
1 tablespoon butter
1 cup medium noodles
2 3/4 cups low-sodium, fat-free vegetable or chicken broth
Salt and pepper to taste

1 In a heavy pot coated with nonstick cooking spray, brown the rice in butter, stirring. Add noodles, broth, and season to taste.

2 Bring mixture to boil, lower heat, simmer, covered, 20–30 minutes, or until rice and noodles are done.

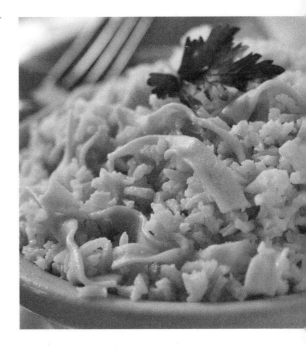

MAKES 6 (3/4-cup) servings
PREP TIME 10 minutes
COOK TIME 30 minutes

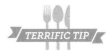
TERRIFIC TIP

Avoid spices such as chili powder, cloves, curry, hot sauces, nutmeg, and pepper. Better tolerated seasonings include herbs such as basil, oregano, and thyme.

. . . .

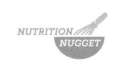
NUTRITION NUGGET

Eat small portions until you start feeling better.

NUTRITIONAL INFORMATION Calories 160, Calories from Fat 13%, Fat 2 g, Saturated Fat 0 g, Cholesterol 6 mg, Sodium 33 mg, Carbohydrates 30 g, Dietary Fiber 1 g, Total Sugars 0 g, Protein 4 g

DIABETIC EXCHANGES 2 starch

LIGHT AND LEMON ANGEL HAIR

Sometimes a tart citrus taste is soothing to the stomach. This light pasta goes easily with whatever you're serving or alone for a comfort pasta dish.

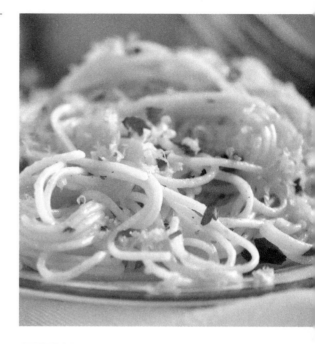

8 ounces angel hair pasta
1/2 teaspoon minced garlic
2 tablespoons olive oil
3 tablespoons lemon juice
1 1/2 teaspoons grated lemon rind, optional
1/3 cup chopped parsley
Salt and pepper to taste

1 Cook pasta according to package directions, reserving 1/4 cup cooking water; drain well and set aside. Transfer pasta to large serving dish.

2 Add remaining ingredients to pasta including reserved 1/4 cup cooking water; toss until well combined. Serve warm or at room temperature.

MAKES 4 (1-cup) servings
PREP TIME 10 minutes
COOK TIME 15 minutes

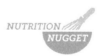

TERRIFIC TIP

If making pasta ahead of time, drizzle and toss with a little olive oil to prevent from sticking together.

. . . .

NUTRITION NUGGET

Even if just a quick sniff, lemons may provide instant relief for nausea symptoms.

NUTRITIONAL INFORMATION Calories 276, Calories from Fat 25%, Fat 8 g, Saturated Fat 1 g, Cholesterol 0 mg, Sodium 9 mg, Carbohydrates 44 g, Dietary Fiber 2 g, Total Sugars 2 g, Protein 8 g

DIABETIC EXCHANGES 3 starch, 1 fat

F D

COUSCOUS AND EDAMAME

Quick cooking couscous and nutritionally packed edamame create a simple soothing side, good at room temperature.

1/2 onion, chopped
1/2 teaspoon minced garlic
2 1/2 cups low-sodium fat-free chicken broth
1 1/2 cups couscous
1 cup shelled edamame, cooked crisp tender according to directions
1 teaspoon ground ginger

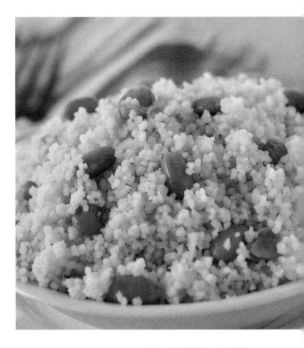

1 In pot coated with nonstick cooking spray, sauté onion and garlic; add chicken broth. Bring to boil and add couscous, cover pot and remove from heat.

2 Let sit 5 minutes, fluff with a fork. Set aside to cool. When cool, stir in edamame and ginger.

MAKES 5 (1-cup) servings
PREP TIME 5 minutes
COOK TIME 5 minutes

TERRIFIC TIP

Couscous is a great grain that is light and easy to digest when not feeling well. Shelled edamame is found with frozen vegetables in the grocery. If using pearl couscous, you will need to cook couscous according to package directions.

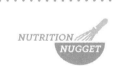

NUTRITION NUGGET

Edamame is an excellent source of protein and adds a nice flavor and crunch. Ginger has anti-nausea properties. For a vegetarian version, use vegetable broth.

NUTRITIONAL INFORMATION Calories 246, Calories from Fat 7%, Fat 2 g, Saturated Fat 0 g, Cholesterol 0 mg, Sodium 263 mg, Carbohydrates 46 g, Dietary Fiber 4 g, Total Sugars 2 g, Protein 10 g

DIABETIC EXCHANGES 3 carbohydrate, 1 very lean protein

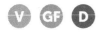

V **GF** **D**

MAKES **4 (1/2-cup) servings**

PREP TIME **10 minutes** | COOK TIME **20 minutes**

RICE PUDDING

Mild, creamy and may be served as a breakfast, snack, or light dessert. Great option for extra rice.

> 1 1/2 cups cooked white rice
> 2 cups skim milk, divided
> 1/4 cup sugar
> Dash salt
> 1 egg, beaten
> 1 teaspoon vanilla extract

1 In medium nonstick pot, combine cooked rice, 1 1/2 cups milk, sugar and salt. Cook over medium heat, stirring, until thick and creamy, 10–15 minutes.

2 In bowl, combine remaining 1/2 cup milk and egg. Gradually pour some of the hot mixture, stirring, into milk-egg mixture. Return to pot. Bring to boil, stirring constantly, and cook until thickened, several minutes. Remove from heat and add vanilla.

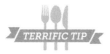

To reheat, stir in milk until creamy consistency—can reheat in microwave. The mixture thickens as it cools.

NUTRITIONAL INFORMATION Calories 188, Calories from Fat 7%, Fat 1 g, Saturated Fat 1 g, Cholesterol 49 mg, Sodium 70 mg, Carbohydrates 36 g, Dietary Fiber 0 g, Total Sugars 19 g, Protein 7 g

DIABETIC EXCHANGES 1 starch, 1/2 fat-free milk, 1 other carbohydrate

---

V **D**

MAKES **4 servings**

PREP TIME **5 minutes** | COOK TIME **5 minutes**

BANANA PUDDING

Pudding makes a satisfying, sweet and simple light dessert or snack.

> 1 (4-serving) package instant banana pudding mix
> 2 cups skim milk
> 2 bananas, diced

1 In a mixing bowl, whisk together pudding mix and milk for 2 minutes. Fold diced bananas into pudding. Transfer to bowls and refrigerate.

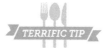

Layer with vanilla wafers and bananas for an old-fashioned banana pudding. Sugar-free pudding may be substituted

. . . .

For extra calories, substitute vanilla nutritional energy drink supplement for skim milk. It's a great way to sneak extra vitamins and calories into your diet. No bananas if you blood counts are low.

NUTRITIONAL INFORMATION Calories 188, Calories from Fat 3%, Fat 1 g, Saturated Fat 0 g, Cholesterol 2 mg, Sodium 435 mg, Carbohydrates 43 g, Dietary Fiber 1 g, Total Sugars 32 g, Protein 5 g

DIABETIC EXCHANGES 1/2 skim milk, 1 fruit, 1 1/2 other carbohydrate

HIGH FIBER

Recipes that are higher in fiber to help relieve constipation.

. . . .

How often do I need to have a bowel movement?

Should I take a stool softener?

Why am I constipated when I have never had this problem before?

Are there any foods that will aid in the relief of my constipation?

. . . .

Constipation can be a problem at any time during your treatment. Certain drugs such as pain medicines and chemotherapy, namely Vincristine, are commonly associated with constipation. Normally, you need to have a bowel movement every forty-eight to seventy-two hours but this will vary among people. You should only be concerned if you notice a difference from your normal routine. Stool softeners such as Colace, Surfak, and Senokot are very helpful. Six to eight glasses of water is extremely important. Bulk forming agents such as Fibercon, Citrucel, or Metamucil will aid your constipation immensely. Laxatives including Milk of Magnesia, Ducolax, Lactulose, Mineral Oil, Magnesium Citrate, in addition to water and a stool softener or bulk forming agent, will alleviate your constipation.

Constipation will decrease your appetite and generally make you feel bad. Foods high in fiber, such as bran, should be a part of your everyday diet. Muffins made with prune juice instead of water can also help with the problem. Fruit salads, vegetable dishes, beans, grains, dried fruit, seeds, raw fruits and vegetables, bread, fruit drinks, figs, raisins, apples, brown rice, pudding and stewed prunes are a few foods which can help keep you regular. If a healthy diet, stool softeners, and laxatives fail, contact your physician. You should not go over seventy-two hours without a bowel movement. The following foods and recipes should really be helpful for you. In addition, drink plenty of fluids throughout the day, eat at regular times, and increase your level of physical activity.

POINTS TO REMEMBER

- Drink 8 to 10 cups of liquid each day, if OK with your doctor. In addition to water, try fluids that have calories like prune juice, warm juices, teas, and hot lemonade.

- Limit drinks and foods that cause gas if it becomes a problem. These include carbonated drinks, broccoli, cabbage, cauliflower, cucumbers, dried beans, peas, and onions.

- Eat high-fiber and bulky foods, such as whole grain breads and cereals, fruits and vegetables (raw and cooked with skins and peels on), popcorn, and dried beans.

- Eat a breakfast that includes a hot drink and high-fiber foods.

- Increase intake of high-fiber foods.

- Try adding 2 tablespoons wheat bran a day to your diet.

- Bran such as wheat bran may be added to baked goods or casseroles. By consuming 2 tablespoons of wheat bran, your stools will be softer and easier to pass. Remember when you increase bran intake; increase your water intake also.

- Add oat or wheat bran to casseroles.

- Choose whole grain cereals and breads.

- Eat more vegetables, raw or cooked.

- Try adding shredded veggies into other casseroles or recipes.

- Do light exercise after eating.

- Try drinking a hot beverage 30 minutes before the usual time for a bowel movement.

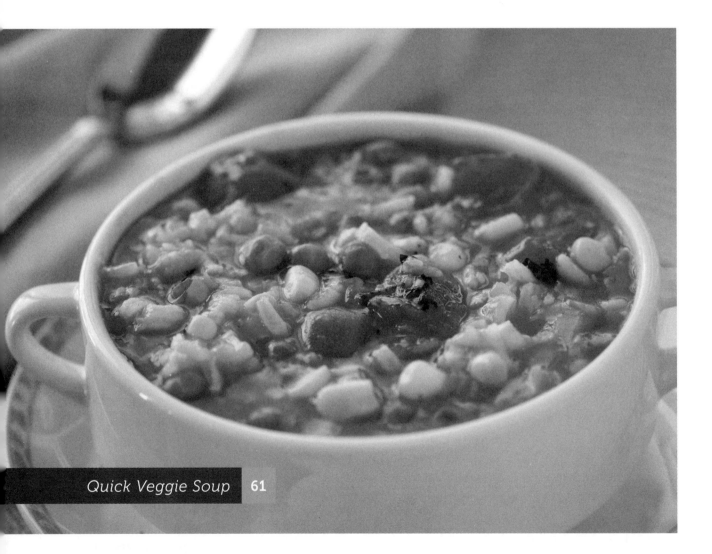

Quick Veggie Soup   61

F V GF D   MAKES **6 (1-cup) servings**

PREP TIME **10 minutes** | COOK TIME **20 minutes**

QUICK VEGGIE SOUP

Here's a speedy recipe for comforting vegetable soup using frozen and canned ingredients.

1/2 cup chopped onion
1 teaspoon minced garlic
3 cups low-sodium fat-free vegetable broth or chicken broth
1 (16-ounce) bag frozen mixed vegetables
1 (14 3/4-ounce) can cream-style corn
1 (14-ounce) can chopped fire-roasted tomatoes
1/4 cup rice
Salt and pepper to taste

1 In large nonstick pot coated with nonstick cooking spray, sauté onion and garlic until tender, about 5 minutes.

2 Add broth, frozen vegetables, cream-style corn, and tomatoes. Bring to boil, add rice and reduce heat; cook 15 minutes. Season to taste.

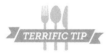

TERRIFIC TIP

Think about adding extra vegetables; either leftovers or whatever you choose. I like fire-roasted tomatoes for their more robust flavor, but you can use any canned tomatoes.

NUTRITIONAL INFORMATION Calories 158, Calories from Fat 5%, Fat 1 g, Saturated Fat 0 g, Cholesterol 0 mg, Sodium 464 mg, Carbohydrates 35 g, Dietary Fiber 5 g, Total Sugars 10 g, Protein 4 g

DIABETIC EXCHANGES 2 starch, 1 vegetable

F V GF   MAKES **8 (1-cup) servings**

PREP TIME **10 minutes** | COOK TIME **20 minutes**

BLACK BEAN SOUP

Take a short-cut with canned beans and southwestern seasoning for an instantaneous super soup.

1 onion, chopped
1 green bell pepper, cored and chopped
1 teaspoon minced garlic
1 (14 1/2-ounce) can chopped fire-roasted tomatoes with juice
1 (4-ounce) can chopped green chilies
1 teaspoon ground cumin
1 teaspoon chili powder
4 (15-ounce) cans black beans, rinsed and drained
4 cups low-sodium fat-free vegetable broth
Salt and pepper to taste

1 In large pot coated with nonstick cooking spray, sauté onion, green pepper, and garlic until tender, 7 minutes. Add remaining ingredients.

2 Remove 2 cups black bean mixture, puree in food processor or blender until smooth.

3 Return pureed mixture to pot with remaining mixture, bring to boil. Lower heat, simmer 10 minutes or until heated. Season to taste.

NUTRITIONAL INFORMATION Calories 212, Calories from Fat 8%, Fat 2 g, Saturated Fat 0 g, Cholesterol 0 mg, Sodium 576 mg, Carbohydrates 34 g, Dietary Fiber 14 g, Total Sugars 3 g, Protein 13 g

DIABETIC EXCHANGES 1/2 skim milk, 1 fruit, 1 1/2 other carbohydrate

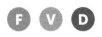

BARLEY SOUP

Terrific twist to basic barley soup made with naturally "sweet" sweet potatoes, earthy mushrooms and carrots.

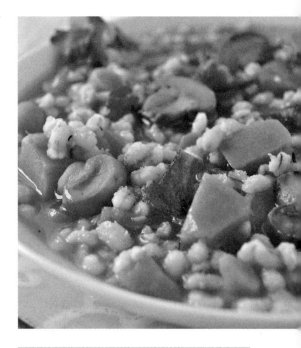

1/2 pound sliced mushrooms
1 teaspoon minced garlic
1 red onion, chopped
1/2 teaspoon dried thyme leaves
8 cups vegetable broth
2 cups chopped carrots
2 cups chopped sweet potatoes, peeled and
  cut into small cubes
3/4 cup medium pearl barley

1 In large nonstick pot coated with nonstick cooking spray, sauté mushrooms, garlic, and onion until tender about 7 minutes.

2 Add thyme, broth, carrots, sweet potatoes and barley. Bring to boil, reduce heat, cover, and cook 25 minutes or until barley and vegetables are tender. Season to taste.

MAKES 11 (1-cup) servings
PREP TIME 10 minutes
COOK TIME 35 minutes

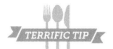

*If soup gets too thick,
add more broth.*

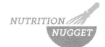

Barley is an excellent source of soluble and insoluble fiber, helping the body metabolize fats and cholesterol along with promoting a healthy digestive tract.

NUTRITIONAL INFORMATION Calories 100, Calories from fat 9%, Fat 1 g, Saturated Fat 1 g, Cholesterol 0 mg, Sodium 52 mg, Carbohydrate 20 g, Dietary Fiber 5 g, Total Sugars 4 g, Protein 5 g

DIABETIC EXCHANGES 1 starch, 1 vegetable

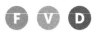

CHUNKY CORN CHOWDER WITH KALE AND SWEET POTATO

I bet you have never had such a fabulous or easier corn chowder with awesome flavor and good nutrition; all in one bowl.

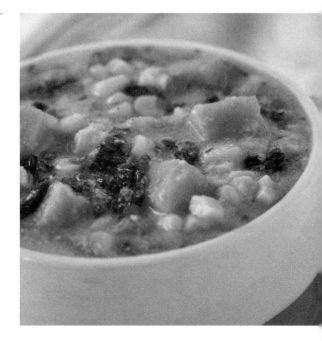

2 tablespoons olive oil
1 onion, diced
1 cup chopped celery
1 teaspoon minced garlic
1/4 cup all-purpose flour
2 cups skim milk
2 cups low-sodium, fat-free vegetable or
  chicken broth
1 (16-ounce) package frozen corn
1 large sweet potato, peeled and cut into
  1/2-inch cubes
Salt and pepper to taste
1 1/2 cups chopped kale

MAKES 8 (1-cup) servings
PREP TIME 15 minutes
COOK TIME 25 minutes

1 In large nonstick pot, heat oil and sauté onion, celery and garlic until tender, 5-7 minutes. Whisk in flour and cook, stirring constantly one minute.

2 Gradually add milk and broth; bring to boil, stirring several minutes or until mixture thickens.

3 Lower heat and add corn and sweet potato, cooking until sweet potato is tender, 6-8 minutes. Season to taste. Before serving stir in kale, cooking several minutes.

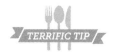

For a thicker soup, dissolve two teaspoons cornstarch in a little water and add. After refrigerating leftovers, if too thick, add more broth. Add rotisserie chicken for a heartier soup.

Keep in your freezer to add nutrition to many dishes, corn is a good source of fiber aiding in digestion, as well as a good source of Vitamin C and other minerals.

NUTRITIONAL INFORMATION Calories 186, Calories from Fat 18%, Fat 4 g, Saturated Fat 1 g, Cholesterol 1 mg, Sodium 91 mg, Carbohydrates 34 g, Dietary Fiber 4 g, Total Sugars 9 g, Protein 6 g

DIABETIC EXCHANGES 2 starch, 1 vegetable, 1/2 fat

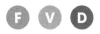

SWEET POTATO CHILI OVER COUSCOUS

Whether you prefer vegetarian or not, this outstanding recipe tops my list! The chili powder, smoky tomatoes, and naturally sweet yams over unassuming couscous are fantastic.

1 tablespoon olive oil

1 onion, chopped

1 red bell pepper, cored and chopped

1 teaspoon minced garlic

1 tablespoon chili powder

1 1/2 pounds sweet potatoes, peeled and cut into 1/2-inch chunks (about 4 cups)

1 (14 1/2-ounce) can fire-roasted diced tomatoes

1 (15-ounce) can dark red kidney beans, rinsed and drained

1 1/2 cups low-sodium fat-free vegetable broth

3 cups cooked couscous

1 In large nonstick pot, heat oil and sauté onion, bell pepper and garlic over medium heat until tender, about 5 minutes. Stir in chili powder for 30 seconds. Add sweet potatoes, tomatoes, beans and broth.

2 Bring to boil, reduce heat, and cook 20–30 minutes or until sweet potatoes are tender. Serve over couscous.

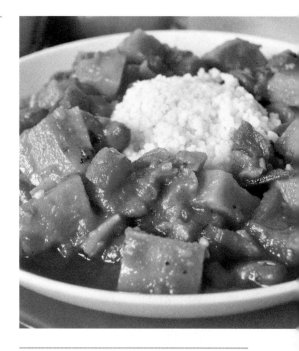

MAKES 6 (1-cup) servings with 1/2 cup couscous

PREP TIME 15 minutes

COOK TIME 30–35 minutes

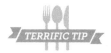

Fire-roasted tomatoes, have a smoky fiery flavor. You can add ground turkey for a heartier version.

With little fat and low in sodium, sweet potatoes provide a delicious dose of fiber and vitamins A, C and E.

NUTRITIONAL INFORMATION Calories 312, Calories from fat 10%, Fat 3 g, Saturated Fat 0 g, Cholesterol 0 mg, Sodium 412 mg, Carbohydrate 60 g, Dietary Fiber 11 g, Total Sugars 12 g, Protein 11 g

DIABETIC EXCHANGES 3 1/2 starch, 2 vegetable

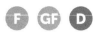

WHITE CHICKEN CHILI

A satisfying warm bowl of my go-to chicken chili with minimal preparation and maximum taste.

1 pound ground chicken
1 onion, chopped
1 teaspoon minced garlic
1 (16-ounce) can white navy beans, rinsed and drained
1 (14-1/2-ounce) can low-sodium fat-free chicken broth
1 (4-ounce) can diced green chilies
2 cups frozen corn
1 teaspoon ground cumin
2 teaspoons chili powder

1 In large nonstick pot, cook chicken, onion, and garlic until chicken is done.

2 Add remaining ingredients and bring to boil. Reduce heat and cook, covered 15 minutes, until heated through.

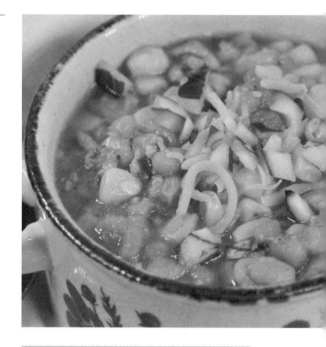

MAKES **8 (1-cup) servings**
PREP TIME **10 minutes**
COOK TIME **25 minutes**

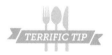

If you prefer, ground turkey may be substituted for ground chicken.

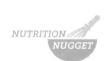

Navy beans are rich in fiber and are a good source of protein.

NUTRITIONAL INFORMATION **Calories 183, Calories from Fat 11%, Fat 2 g, Saturated Fat 0 g, Cholesterol 36 mg, Sodium 378 mg, Carbohydrates 24 g, Dietary Fiber 5 g, Total Sugars 4 g, Protein 18 g**

DIABETIC EXCHANGES **1 1/2 starch, 2 lean meat**

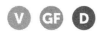

BLACK BEAN AND CORN SALAD

Fast and fantastic, black beans, corn and tomatoes with a little lemon will perk up those taste buds.

1 (15-ounce) can black beans, rinsed and drained
1 1/2 cups frozen corn, thawed
1 tomato, chopped
1/4 cup fresh cilantro, chopped, optional
1/4 cup chopped red onion
3 tablespoons lemon juice
2 tablespoons olive oil
Salt and pepper to taste

1 In large bowl, combine all ingredients. Refrigerate until ready to serve.

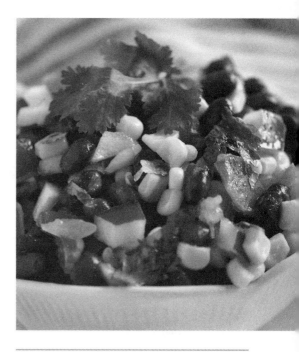

MAKES 6 (1/2-cup) servings

PREP TIME 5 minutes

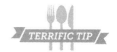
TERRIFIC TIP

A great side to chicken or fish and also may be used as a dip.

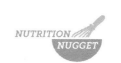
NUTRITION NUGGET

Rinsing and draining canned beans can reduce your sodium content by 40%.

NUTRITIONAL INFORMATION Calories 148, Calories from Fat 32%, Fat 5 g, Saturated Fat 1 g, Cholesterol 0 mg, Sodium 204 mg, Carbohydrates 21 g, Dietary Fiber 5 g, Total Sugars 3 g, Protein 5 g

DIABETIC EXCHANGES 1 1/2 starch, 1 fat

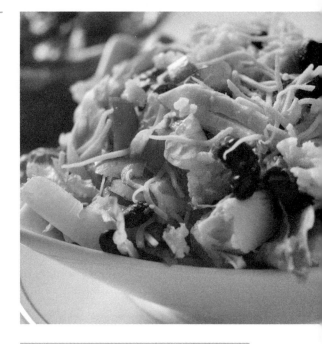

CHICKEN TACO RICE SALAD

A favorite toss-together southwestern style chef salad with simple ingredients and big flavor.

1 (5-ounce) package yellow rice
6 cups mixed salad greens
2 cups skinless rotisserie chicken, shredded
1 (15-ounce) can black beans, rinsed and drained
1 cup grape or cherry tomato halves
1/2 cup chopped red onion
1/2 cup shredded, reduced-fat sharp Cheddar cheese

1 Prepare rice according to package directions. Cool; set aside.

2 In large bowl, combine cooled rice and all ingredients. Toss with Salsa Vinaigrette.

SALSA VINAIGRETTE

Salsa with a few ingredients makes a great-tasting vinaigrette. Use whatever needed and save extra for another time.

1 cup salsa
2 teaspoons chili powder
1/2 teaspoon ground cumin
1 tablespoon lime juice
2 tablespoons olive oil

1 In small bowl, whisk together all ingredients.

MAKES 6 (2-cup) servings of salad with Salsa Vinaigrette

PREP TIME 10 minutes

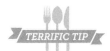
TERRIFIC TIP

Rotisserie chicken is an easy time-saving way to add tasty lean protein to dishes saving you a step. To cut sodium and add nutrition, use brown rice.

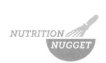
NUTRITION NUGGET

Think of beans as the nutritional crouton, sprinkle on salads or in casseroles and soups to boost your fiber intake.

NUTRITIONAL INFORMATION Calories 327, Calories from Fat 29%, Fat 11 g, Saturated Fat 3 g, Cholesterol 57 mg, Sodium 923 mg, Carbohydrates 36 g, Dietary Fiber 6 g, Total Sugars 4 g, Protein 23 g

DIABETIC EXCHANGES 2 starch, 1 vegetable, 2 1/2 lean meat

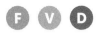

BAKED BEANS

A different twist to a traditional dish—a remarkable recipe!

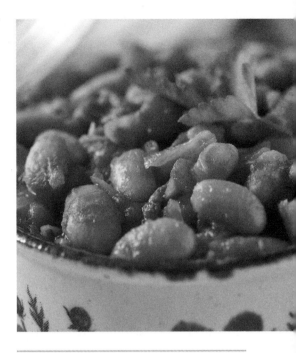

1 onion, chopped
1 1/2 teaspoons minced garlic
1 cup light beer or diet cola
1 (15 1/2-ounce) can tomato sauce
3 tablespoons light brown sugar
2 tablespoons balsamic vinegar
1 tablespoon Dijon mustard
3 (15 1/2-ounce) cans cannellini or great Northern beans, rinsed and drained

1 Preheat oven 350°F. Coat 2-quart baking dish with nonstick cooking spray.

2 In large nonstick pot, sauté onion and garlic; cook until tender, 5–7 minutes. Add remaining ingredients except beans. Bring to boil, reduce heat, and cook 5 minutes.

3 Add beans, stirring to mix well. Transfer to baking dish and bake, covered, 35–40 minutes.

MAKES **16 (1/2 cup) servings**
PREP TIME **10 minutes**
COOK TIME **45 minutes**

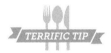
TERRIFIC TIP

If you want you can toss in some cooked turkey bacon pieces.

DOC'S NOTE

A nutritional bargain, beans provide an excellent source of fiber and folate, helping with digestive health and weight maintenance.

NUTRITIONAL INFORMATION Calories 91, Calories from Fat 0%, Fat 0 g, Saturated Fat 0 g, Cholesterol 0 mg, Sodium 338 mg, Carbohydrates 17 g, Dietary Fiber 3 g, Total Sugars 4 g, Protein 4 g

DIABETIC EXCHANGES **1 starch**

TASTY KALE AND WHITE BEANS

Never cooked kale before? This recipe truly knocked it out of the park when featured on WebMD website!

1/3 cup diced Canadian bacon
1 tablespoon olive oil
1 onion, chopped
6 cups chopped kale
1 (15-ounce) can Great northern beans,
 rinsed and drained
1 cup low-sodium fat-free chicken broth
Salt and pepper to taste

1 In large nonstick skillet coated with nonstick cooking spray over medium heat, cook Canadian bacon until golden brown, several minutes. Add oil and onion, sauté until tender, about 5 minutes.

2 Add kale, beans and broth and cook, stirring, about 10 minutes or until kale is tender. Season to taste.

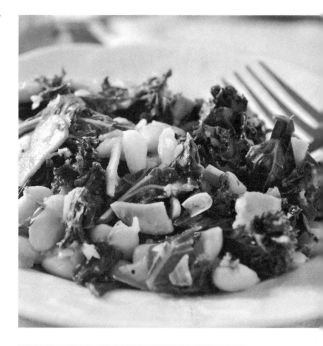

MAKES **6 servings**
PREP TIME **10 minutes**
COOK TIME **15 minutes**

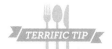

Look for packages of already chopped kale. Omit Canadian bacon, if desired.

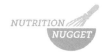

Keep kale a part of your regular menu as only 1 cup provides a good source of fiber, 15% of your daily calcium recommended intake, 180% of vitamin A, and 200% of vitamin C!

NUTRITIONAL INFORMATION Calories 137, Calories from Fat 21%, Fat 3 g, Saturated Fat 1 g, Cholesterol 4 mg, Sodium 234 mg, Carbohydrates 20 g, Dietary Fiber 6 g, Total Sugars 2 g, Protein 8 g

DIABETIC EXCHANGES 1/2 starch, 2 vegetable, 1/2 lean meat

V **GF**

EGGPLANT PARMESAN

Here's a quick and easy version of this classic popular Italian dish.

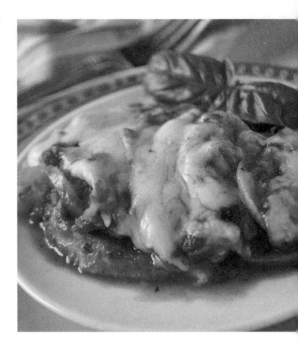

- 2 medium eggplants, peeled and cut in 1/2-inch slices (about 1 1/2 pounds)
- 2 onions, thinly sliced into rings
- 1 (26-ounce) jar healthy marinara sauce
- 1 teaspoon dried oregano leaves
- 1 teaspoon dried basil leaves
- 1 1/2 cups shredded part-skim mozzarella cheese

1. Preheat oven 350°F. Coat oblong 2-quart baking dish with nonstick cooking spray.

2. Arrange eggplant slices along bottom of dish. Top with onions.

3. In bowl, mix marinara sauce, oregano and basil. Spread evenly over onion slices.

4. Bake 40–45 minutes or until eggplant is tender. Sprinkle with mozzarella cheese and return to oven 10 minutes longer or until cheese is melted.

MAKES **6 servings**
PREP TIME **15 minutes**
COOK TIME **50 minutes**

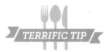
TERRIFIC TIP

Serve with angel hair pasta. Eggplant is very filling, supplying few calories, high in fiber and virtually no fat.

· · · · · · · · · · · · · · ·

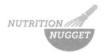
NUTRITION
NUGGET

Unlike most vitamins in fresh fruits and vegetables, the antioxidant lycopene, found in tomatoes, especially canned, actually improves with the cooking process instead of diminishing it.

NUTRITIONAL INFORMATION Calories 182, Calories from Fat 29%, Fat 6 g, Saturated Fat 3 g, Cholesterol 18 mg, Sodium 519 mg, Carbohydrates 24 g, Dietary Fiber 8 g, Total Sugars 16 g, Protein 10 g

DIABETIC EXCHANGES 1 starch, 2 vegetable, 1 lean meat

F **V** **GF**

SOUTHWESTERN RICE

Turn leftover rice into a meatless entrée or a hearty family pleasing side; this recipe is as simple as opening cans.

2 cups cooked rice
1 (15-ounce) can corn, drained (or frozen corn)
1 (15-ounce) can black beans, rinsed and drained
1 (10-ounce) can tomatoes and green chilies
2 cups shredded reduced-fat Mexican blend cheese, divided
1 bunch green onions, chopped (reserving 2 tablespoons)
1 (2 1/4-ounce) can sliced black olives, drained
1 cup nonfat sour cream

1 Preheat oven 350°F. Coat 2-quart oblong baking dish with nonstick cooking spray.

2 Combine all ingredients using 1 3/4 cups cheese in prepared dish. Bake 45–50 minutes. Remove from oven and sprinkle with remaining 1/4 cup cheese and remaining 2 tablespoons green onions. Return to oven 5 minutes or until cheese is melted.

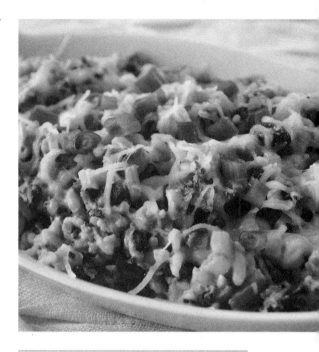

MAKES **8 (1-cup) servings**
PREP TIME **10 minutes**
COOK TIME **55 minutes**

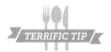
TERRIFIC TIP

Put mixture into a wrap for a mouthwatering meatless meal.

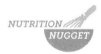
NUTRITION NUGGET

Give brown rice a try for a nutritional boost.
1 cup white rice = 1 g fiber
1 cup brown rice = 3 g fiber

NUTRITIONAL INFORMATION Calories 269, Calories from Fat 23%, Fat 7 g, Saturated Fat 3 g, Cholesterol 23 mg, Sodium 720 mg, Carbohydrates 38 g, Dietary Fiber 5 g, Total Sugars 5 g, Protein 14 g

DIABETIC EXCHANGES 2 1/2 starch, 1 1/2 lean meat

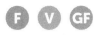

SOUTHWESTERN BAKED SWEET POTATOES

Layers of flavors explode into an exceptionally delicious sweet potato with a cool yogurt sauce and black bean topping.

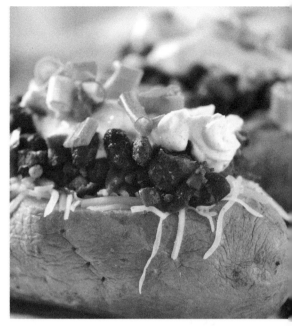

4 medium sized sweet potatoes
1/2 cup nonfat plain Greek yogurt
1 1/2 teaspoons chili powder, divided
1 teaspoon ground cumin, divided
Dash salt
1 teaspoon olive oil
1/2 red onion, diced
1 red bell pepper, cored and diced
1/2 teaspoon paprika
1 (15-ounce) can black beans, rinsed and drained
1/2 cup reduced-fat shredded Mexican cheese blend
1/4 cup chopped green onions

1 Poke holes in sweet potato with fork. Microwave potatoes 8-10 minutes or until soft and cooked through.

2 In small bowl, mix together yogurt, 1/2 teaspoon chili powder, 1/2 teaspoon cumin, and salt; set aside.

3 In small nonstick skillet, heat oil and sauté onion, bell pepper, remaining 1 teaspoon chili powder, remaining 1/2 teaspoon cumin and paprika until onion is slightly caramelized, about 5 minutes. Stir in black beans until heated.

4 Cut thin slice off top of potato and open wider by squeezing potato. Top each potato with cheese, black bean mixture, yogurt mixture and green onions.

MAKES 4 potatoes
PREP TIME 15 minutes
COOK TIME 15 minutes

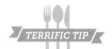

If desired bake potatoes in oven at 400°F. about 1 hour. For smaller portions, cut potatoes in half and fill each half.

. . . .

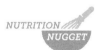

Makes a wonderful vegetarian meal or a hearty side.

NUTRITIONAL INFORMATION Calories 372, Calories from Fat 12%, Fat 5 g, Saturated Fat 2 g, Cholesterol 9 mg, Sodium 567 mg, Carbohydrates 66 g, Dietary Fiber 14 g, Total Sugars 13 g, Protein 16 g

DIABETIC EXCHANGES 4 starch, 1 vegetable, 1 lean meat

F **V** **GF** **D**

BUTTERNUT SQUASH, BLACK BEAN AND FETA ENCHILADAS
WITH SALSA VERDE

Six ingredient vegetarian enchiladas burst with flavor and effortless to make.

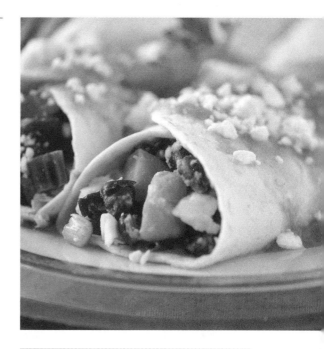

4 cups peeled butternut squash
1 (15-ounce) can black beans, rinsed and drained
1 bunch green onions, chopped
3/4 cup crumbled reduced-fat feta cheese, divided
2 cups salsa verde
8 large corn or flour tortillas

1 Preheat oven 400°F. Coat baking pan with foil and coat with nonstick cooking spray.

2 Place squash on prepared pan. Bake 20–25 minutes or until squash is tender but not mushy.

3 Reduce heat to 350°F. In bowl, combine cooked squash, black beans, green onions, and 1/2 cup feta.

4 Coat 3-quart oblong baking dish with nonstick cooking spray and spread a little of the salsa verde on the bottom. Fill tortillas with about 1/2 cup filling, rolling up and place seam side down in dish. Pour remaining sauce over enchiladas. Sprinkle remaining cheese over sauce.

5 Cover pan with foil and bake 20 minutes or until thoroughly heated.

MAKES **8 enchiladas**
PREP TIME **20 minutes**
COOK TIME **45 minutes**

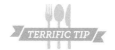

Roasted vegetables are easy to prepare with easy clean-up, and more flavorful. Look for pre-cut butternut squash in grocery.

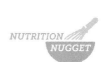

Make this recipe gluten-free with corn tortillas.

NUTRITIONAL INFORMATION Calories 202, Calories from Fat 13%, Fat 3 g, Saturated Fat 1 g, Cholesterol 5 mg, Sodium 539 mg, Carbohydrates 36 g, Dietary Fiber 7 g, Total Sugars 7 g, Protein 8 g

DIABETIC EXCHANGES 2 starch, 1 vegetable, 1 lean meat

SHRIMP TOSS WITH ASPARAGUS AND WHITE BEANS

A trouble-free toss together dish with shrimp, asparagus and white beans in a light sauce. Serve over pasta and sprinkle with Parmesan cheese. Use low-sodium tomatoes to make recipe diabetic.

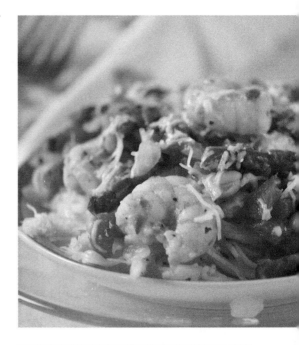

1 tablespoon olive oil
1 pound asparagus, cut into 1 inch pieces
1 tablespoon minced garlic
1 pound medium shrimp, peeled
1 (14-ounce) can fire-roasted tomatoes, drained
1 (15-ounce) can navy beans, rinsed and drained
1 cup low-sodium, fat-free chicken broth
2 teaspoons cornstarch
1/2 teaspoon dried basil leaves
Salt and pepper to taste
Grated Parmesan cheese, optional

MAKES 4 (1 1/4-cups) servings
PREP TIME 10 minutes
COOK TIME 15 minutes

1 In large nonstick skillet, heat oil and cook asparagus and garlic 1–2 minutes, stirring.

2 Add shrimp and cook until almost done, 3–5 minutes. Add tomatoes and beans, stirring.

3 In small bowl, mix together broth and cornstarch, stir into skillet. Cook over medium heat until thickened, stirring frequently. Add basil, season to taste and sprinkle with cheese if desired.

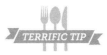

TERRIFIC TIP

Chicken may be substituted for the shrimp. If using chicken, cook chicken first in skillet in oil and proceed with recipe adding asparagus.

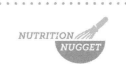

NUTRITION NUGGET

Asparagus provides a great source of vitamins A, B6, C, E, and folacin. Beans provide fiber, iron, and vitamin C.

NUTRITIONAL INFORMATION Calories 287, Calories from Fat 16%, Fat 5 g, Saturated Fat 1 g, Cholesterol 143 mg, Sodium 931 mg, Carbohydrates 34 g, Dietary Fiber 9 g, Total Sugars 7 g, Protein 27 g

DIABETIC EXCHANGES 1 1/2 starch, 2 vegetable, 3 lean meat

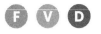

PREP TIME 10 minutes | COOK TIME 20 minutes

PREP TIME 5 minutes

HONEY BRAN MUFFINS

A fiber filled honey bran muffin makes a great quick breakfast or snack on the go.

- 2 cups wheat bran
- 2 cups all-purpose flour
- 1 teaspoon baking soda
- 1/2 cup light brown sugar
- 3 eggs
- 1 cup prune juice
- 1/2 cup canola oil or applesauce
- 1/2 cup honey
- 1 cup raisins

1 Preheat oven 400°F.

2 In bowl, combine bran, flour, baking soda, and brown sugar. Add eggs, prune juice, oil, and honey, mixing well. Stir in raisins. Pour batter into paper lined muffin tins. Bake 20 minutes.

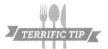
TERRIFIC TIP

Muffins are great to keep in the freezer for a quick snack or breakfast. Try adding nuts.

NUTRITIONAL INFORMATION Calories 219, Calories from Fat 28%, Fat 7 g, Saturated Fat 1 g, Cholesterol 35 mg, Sodium 103 mg, Carbohydrates 38 g, Dietary Fiber 4 g, Total Sugars 21 g, Protein 4 g

DIABETIC EXCHANGES 1 starch, 1 other carbohydrate, 1/2 fruit, 1 fat

ALL NATURAL LAXATIVE

This is not a flavor savor but it works. Always drink fluids to increase the effectiveness of the fiber.

- 1 1/4 cups unprocessed bran
- 1 cup prune juice
- 1 tablespoon molasses or honey
- 1 cup applesauce

1 Mix all ingredients and store in covered container in refrigerator up to 7 days.

2 Stir before taking. Take 2 tablespoons every night as needed.

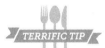
TERRIFIC TIP

If 2 tablespoons causes diarrhea, decrease to 1 tablespoon. If you find that 2 tablespoons is not enough, you can increase to 3 or 4 tablespoons. If this combination is not working, you can also take a laxative.

DOC'S NOTE

The prune juice comes in 6 packs of (5 1/2-ounce) cans. The high fiber content acts by drawing water into the colon, softening your stool and aiding in bowel movements.

NUTRITIONAL INFORMATION Calories 28, Calories from Fat 0%, Fat 0 g, Saturated Fat 0 g, Cholesterol 0 mg, Sodium 1 mg, Carbohydrates 7 g, Dietary Fiber 2 g, Total Sugars 4 g, Protein 1 g

DIABETIC EXCHANGES 1/2 fruit

SORE MOUTH OR THROAT

Maintain nutrition with soft, soothing recipes that ease chewing and swallowing for a dry, sore mouth and throat.

I have no appetite. Is there anything to help me?

Should I eat hot or cold foods?

What foods should I eat?

. . . .

Your mouth normally will get sore 7–10 days following certain chemotherapy treatments. Remember to do your mouth care: 1 teaspoon baking soda, 1 teaspoon salt in a quart of tap water. Rinse and spit after each meal. Make a fresh solution each morning and discard at the end of the day. Try eating soft or puréed foods. Use a straw for all liquids or puréed foods. This is a good time to use plastic utensils to avoid the metallic taste. Eating foods at room temperature or cool are easier to handle when your mouth is sore. Raw foods tend to irritate your mouth and should be avoided.

If you are still losing ground, talk to your physicians about the following appetite stimulants:

1. Liquid Megace—800 mg/day × 30 days then decrease to 400 mg/day.

2. Megace—40 mg twice per day and Marinol 2.5 mg by mouth twice per day.

Remember, if you find one food that you can tolerate do not hesitate to eat it repeatedly. The mouth soreness is usually associated with a low white blood cell count. As soon as your counts rise, the soreness will resolve. Cephacol, Xylocaine, and pain medicines are sometimes needed to ease the mouth pain. Sometimes patients take a pain pill 30 minutes prior to meals to allow them to eat. If you have obvious sores on your lips,

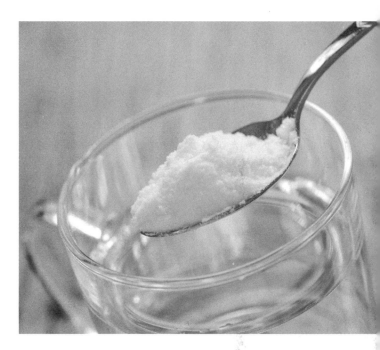

a small amount of vitamin E can sometimes help. Puncture a 500 unit vitamin E capsule and squeeze the contents on the ulcer 3 times per day.

If you have these problems, eating soft, bland foods and lukewarm or cool foods can be soothing. On the other hand, foods that are coarse, dry, or scratchy should be avoided. In addition, you may find that tart, salty or acidic fruits and juices, alcohol, and spicy foods may be irritating and should be avoided. Rinsing your mouth regularly with one teaspoon of baking soda and eight ounces of water or salt water can help prevent infections and improve healing.

POINTS TO REMEMBER

- Avoid tart, acidic, or salty foods and drinks such as citrus fruit juices (grapefruit, orange, lime), pickled and vinegary foods, tomato-based foods, and some canned broths.

- Avoid rough-textured foods, such as dry toast, granola, and raw fruits and vegetables.

- Eat food that is cool or room temperature. Very hot or cold foods can cause discomfort.

- Limit alcohol, caffeine, and tobacco. These substances can dry out your mouth and throat and promote further irritation.

- Avoid spices such as chili powder, cloves, curry, hot sauces, nutmeg, and pepper.

- Season foods with herbs such as basil, oregano, and thyme.

- Softer and easy to swallow foods include cream soups, cheeses, mashed potatoes, pastas, yogurt, eggs, custards, puddings, cooked cereals, ice cream, casseroles, gravies, syrups, breakfast-type recipes, milkshakes, and nutritional liquid food supplements.

- Use a straw for liquids.

- Try chewing sugar-free gum or suck on sugar-free candies.

- Cut food into small pieces.

- Practice good oral hygiene.

- Use oral anesthetics such as ulcerease. Ask your doctor for a "stomatitis (sore mouth) cocktail."

- Xylocaine—equal parts; Maalox—equal parts; Benadryl—equal parts. Swish and swallow one teaspoon every four hours as needed for pain.

SOME SOFT FOODS TO INCLUDE:

- Scrambled eggs

- Applesauce, bananas, watermelon, and other soft fruits.

- Cottage cheese, milk shakes, or smoothies.

- Puddings, flavored gelatin.

- Cooked cereals such as oatmeal or cream of wheat.

- Mashed potatoes or sweet potatoes, macaroni and cheese, or mashed vegetables.

(V) (GF) (D)

GINGER TEA

Treat yourself to an invigorating cup of ginger tea with this easy, tasty recipe. The secret to making really flavorful ginger tea is to use lots of ginger (more than you think you will need) and I like to add a little lime juice and honey.

4–6 thin slices raw peeled ginger
1 1/2–2 cups water
1 tablespoon lemon or lime juice or to taste
1–2 tablespoons honey or to taste, optional

1. In small pot, bring ginger and water to boil, lower heat, cover, and simmer at least 10-15 minutes. For stronger and tangier tea, boil 20 minutes or more, and use more slices of ginger.

2. Remove from heat and add lemon juice and honey to taste.

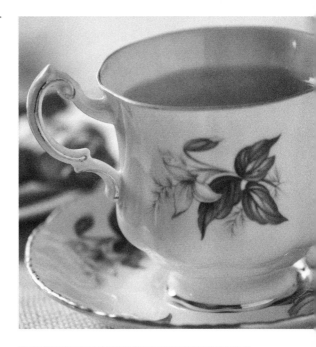

MAKES 1 servings
PREP TIME 5 minutes
COOK TIME 15 minutes

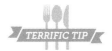
TERRIFIC TIP

Use a peeler to remove skin off ginger.

. . . .

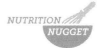
NUTRITION NUGGET

Ginger is an immune boosting root, long believed to have medicinal properties—helping with nausea and upset stomach, also having anti-inflammatory benefits.

NUTRITIONAL INFORMATION Calories 3, Calories from Fat 0%, Fat 0 g, Saturated Fat 0 g, Cholesterol 0 mg, Sodium 11 mg, Carbohydrates 1 g, Dietary Fiber 0 g, Total Sugars 0 g, Protein 8 g

DIABETIC EXCHANGES Free

PREP TIME 5 minutes | **COOK TIME** 5 minutes

PREP TIME 5 minutes | **COOK TIME** 10 minutes

APPLESAUCE OATMEAL

Start your day off with this easy to eat recipe that takes oatmeal to a new level.

1 cup skim milk
3/4 cup old-fashioned oatmeal
1/2 cup unsweetened applesauce
1 tablespoon light brown sugar
1/8 teaspoon ground cinnamon

1 In small nonstick pot, bring milk to a boil. Add oatmeal and reduce heat. Cook about 5 minutes or until thickened, stirring occasionally.

2 Add applesauce, brown sugar, and cinnamon, stirring until well mixed. Serve immediately.

TERRIFIC TIP

Instead of applesauce, try stirring in a mashed banana for banana oatmeal and, if your mouth isn't sore, add some raisins.

WEIGHT GAIN PANCAKES

Whole milk can be used instead of the drink supplement, if desired. Top with fresh fruit or sliced bananas for added nutrition if feeling better, but make sure no citrus fruit.

1/2 cup pancake and waffle mix
1/2 cup vanilla nutritional drink supplement
1 egg
1 tablespoon canola oil

1 In large bowl, whisk together all ingredients just until combined. Let stand 1-2 minutes.

2 Heat large nonstick skillet coated with nonstick cooking spray over medium heat. Using 1/4 cup batter per pancake, cook pancakes 1–2 minutes on each side or until lightly browned. Recoat pan between pancakes.

DOC'S NOTE

The nutritional drink supplement supplies essential vitamins and minerals, plus high quality protein and carbohydrates for energy, making it a great way to use as added value for milk in recipes.

NUTRITIONAL INFORMATION Calories 206, Calories from Fat 9%, Fat 2 g, Saturated Fat 1 g, Cholesterol 2 mg, Sodium 68 mg, Carbohydrates 40 g, Dietary Fiber 4 g, Total Sugars 19 g, Protein 9 g

DIABETIC EXCHANGES 1 1/2 starch, 1/2 fruit, 1/2 skim milk, 1/2 other carbohydrate

NUTRITIONAL INFORMATION Calories 80, Calories from Fat 39%, Fat 3 g, Saturated Fat 1 g, Cholesterol 32 mg, Sodium 131 mg, Carbohydrates 10 g, Dietary Fiber 0 g, Total Sugars 2 g, Protein 3 g

DIABETIC EXCHANGES 1/2 starch, 1/2 fat

F **V**

CHEESE GRITS

Ever had grits? Give this tasty, easy to make and easy to swallow recipe a try!

2 cups low-sodium fat-free chicken broth
1 1/2 cups skim milk
1 cup quick grits
1 cup shredded reduced-fat Cheddar cheese

1 In nonstick pot, bring broth and milk to boil. Add grits, reduce heat, cook about 5 minutes, stirring occasionally. Add cheese; stir until cheese melts.

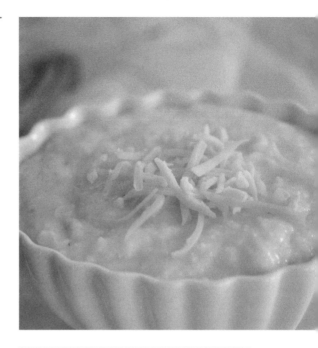

MAKES 6 servings
PREP TIME 5 minutes
COOK TIME 10 minutes

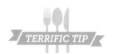
TERRIFIC TIP

If not eating immediately or if reheating, you may need to add more milk to make creamy.

· · · · · · · · · · · · · · · · ·

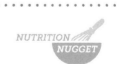
NUTRITION
NUGGET

For weight gain, don't use reduced-fat products or add in powdered milk.

NUTRITIONAL INFORMATION Calories 175, Calories from Fat 20%, Fat 4 g, Saturated Fat 2 g, Cholesterol 11 mg, Sodium 175 mg, Total Carbohydrate 24 g, Dietary Fiber 0 g, Total Sugars 3 g, Protein 10 g

DIABETIC EXCHANGES 1 1/2 starch, 1 lean meat

AVOCADO CUCUMBER SOUP

Buttery avocados and cucumbers pair together in this creamy chilled soup.

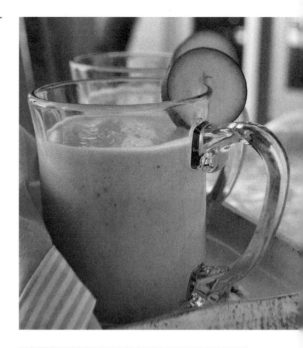

1 large avocado, peeled, pitted, and halved
2 cucumbers, peeled, seeded, and halved
1 cup vegetable broth or low-sodium
  fat-free chicken
1 cup fat-free evaporated skimmed milk
2 tablespoons lemon juice
Salt and pepper to taste

1 In blender or food processor, blend avocado, cucumbers, broth, evaporated milk, and lemon juice until smooth. Season to taste. Refrigerate, covered, until chilled.

2 If soup is too thick, gradually add more broth or evaporated milk.

MAKES 6 (3/4-cup) servings
PREP TIME 5 minutes

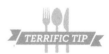

TERRIFIC TIP

To easily seed cucumbers, cut in half and run a knife or spoon down the center of cucumber to scrape out seeds.

· · · · · · · · · · · · · · · · ·

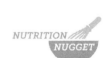

NUTRITION NUGGET

Avocados contain healthy unsaturated fats that help your body absorb and use vitamins, as well as help to maintain cell membranes.

NUTRITIONAL INFORMATION Calories 99, Calories from fat 46%, Fat 5 g, Saturated Fat 1 g, Cholesterol 2 mg, Sodium 64 mg, Carbohydrate 10 g, Dietary Fiber 3 g, Total Sugars 7 g, Protein 5 g

DIABETIC EXCHANGES 1 vegetable, 1/2 fat-free milk, 1 fat

F **V**

EASY POTATO SOUP

Starting with frozen hash browns means no peeling potatoes for an incredibly marvelous, yet simple soup.

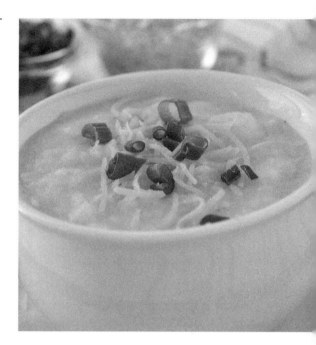

6 cups frozen hash brown potatoes, partially thawed
6 cups fat-free chicken or vegetable broth
1 onion, chopped
1/4 cup all-purpose flour
1 (12-ounce) can evaporated skimmed milk, divided
3/4 cup nonfat plain Greek yogurt
Salt and pepper to taste
Green onions, cheese, optional toppings

1 In large nonstick pot, combine hash browns, broth, and onion; bring to boil, reduce heat, and cook, covered, 8–10 minutes.

2 In small bowl, whisk together flour with 1/3 cup evaporated milk. Add to potato mixture with remaining milk. Bring to boil, reduce heat, and cook, stirring, 5 minutes or until thickened.

3 Remove from heat and stir in yogurt; don't boil after adding, stirring until well combined. Season to taste and sprinkle with toppings, if desired.

MAKES 8 (1-cup) servings
PREP TIME 5 minutes
COOK TIME 20 minutes

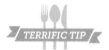
TERRIFIC TIP

I like using Greek yogurt as it is richer, and creamier. If you feel better, you can add condiments such as green onions, turkey bacon or cheese.

· · · · · · · · · · · · · · · · ·

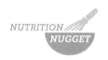
NUTRITION NUGGET

Greek yogurt is higher in calcium than plain yogurt.

NUTRITIONAL INFORMATION Calories 256, Calories from Fat 2%, Fat 1 g, Saturated Fat 0 g, Cholesterol 2 mg, Sodium 1051 mg, Carbohydrates 51 g, Dietary Fiber 4 g, Total Sugars 10 g, Protein 13 g

DIABETIC EXCHANGES 3 starch, 1/2 fat-free milk

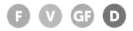

CAULIFLOWER SOUP

I saw a big head of fresh cauliflower at the grocery store and was inspired to create this tantalizing delicious soothing soup.

2 tablespoons olive oil
1 onion, finely chopped
1 large cauliflower, broken into florets (about 8 cups)
1 1/2 teaspoons ground turmeric
1 teaspoon ground cumin
1 tablespoon minced garlic
1 large potato, peeled and diced (about 1 1/2 cups)
3 cups fat-free vegetable broth
1 cup skim milk

1 In large nonstick pot coated with nonstick cooking spray, heat oil and sauté onion over medium heat until tender. Add cauliflower, turmeric, cumin and garlic; stir about 5 minutes.

2 Add potato and vegetable broth. Bring to boil, reduce heat and simmer about 15 minutes or until cauliflower is tender.

3 In blender, food processor or with hand-held blender, puree until smooth. Add milk and simmer 5 minutes or until heated.

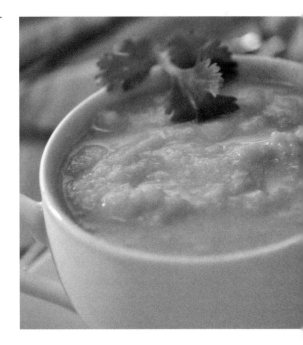

MAKES 8 (1-cup) servings
PREP TIME 10 minutes
COOK TIME 30 minutes

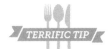

A hand-held blender is a useful kitchen tool to cream soups and smoothies with easy clean up.

· · · · · · · · · · · · · · · · ·

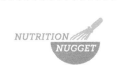

Turmeric is a bright yellow spice that has shown to have antioxidant and anti-inflammatory properties.

NUTRITIONAL INFORMATION Calories 103, Calories from Fat 31%, Fat 4 g, Saturated Fat 1 g, Cholesterol 1 mg, Sodium 398 mg, Carbohydrates 15 g, Dietary Fiber 3 g, Total Sugars 6 g, Protein 4 g

DIABETIC EXCHANGES 1 1/2 starch, 2 vegetable, 1/2 fat

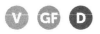

WATERMELON AND CANTALOUPE SALAD

Cool crisp watermelon and refreshing cantaloupe, with mint and fresh basil create an extraordinary and invigorating salad.

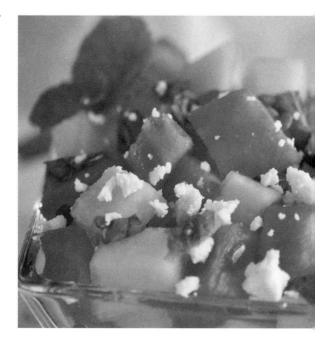

2 cups watermelon small chunks or balls
1 cup cantaloupe small chunks or balls
2 tablespoons lemon juice
2 tablespoons honey
2 tablespoons chopped fresh mint
2 teaspoons dried basil leaves or 1 teaspoon chopped fresh basil
Salt and pepper to taste
1/4 cup reduced-fat feta cheese

1 In large bowl, combine watermelon and cantaloupe.

2 In small bowl, mix together lemon juice, honey, mint and basil. Season to taste. Toss with watermelon mixture. Refrigerate until serving. Add feta before serving.

MAKES 6 (1/2-cup) servings
PREP TIME 15 minutes

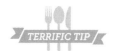

You can make this salad the night before as the flavors meld together.

· · · · · · · · · · · · · · · · ·

This salad is packed with immune-boosting carotenoid antioxidants found in watermelon and cantaloupe.

NUTRITIONAL INFORMATION Calories 60, Calories from fat 11%, Fat 1 g, Saturated Fat 0 g, Cholesterol 2 mg, Sodium 89 mg, Carbohydrates 13 g, Dietary Fiber 1 g, Total Sugars 11 g, Protein 2 g

DIABETIC EXCHANGES 1 fruit

F D

CHICKEN POT PIE

By cutting chicken and sweet potatoes into small pieces, this nutritious quick and classic dish will be easier to eat.

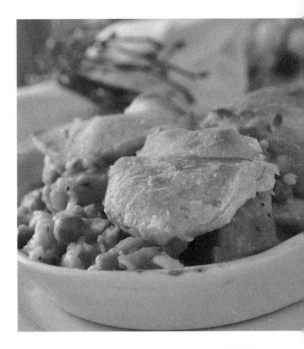

1 pound boneless skinless chicken breasts, cut into very small pieces
Salt and pepper to taste
4 tablespoons all-purpose flour
2 cups low-sodium fat-free chicken broth
1/2 cup diced peeled sweet potatoes
1 teaspoon dried thyme leaves
2 cups frozen mixed vegetables
5 flaky refrigerator biscuits

1 Preheat oven 400°F. Coat pie plate or ramekins with nonstick cooking spray.

2 In nonstick skillet coated with nonstick cooking spray, cook chicken breasts over medium heat 5–7 minutes or until brown. Season to taste.

3 Add flour and gradually add broth, stirring and cooking over medium heat until bubbly. Add sweet potatoes and thyme; bring to boil, stirring, about 5 minutes.

4 Add mixed vegetables, cooking another 5 minutes until vegetables and sweet potato are tender. Transfer chicken mixture to prepared dish. Split biscuits into layers and cover top. Bake 10–12 minutes or until the pastry is golden brown.

MAKES 6 (2/3-cup) servings
PREP TIME 10 minutes
COOK TIME 25 minutes

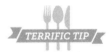

Save time with leftover or rotisserie chicken. Cut chicken into very small pieces and vegetables are already in small pieces to help with swallowing.

· · · · · · · · · · · · · · · · · ·

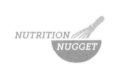

This is a complete meal. Carrots and sweet potatoes provide beta carotene and fiber while celery is rich in vitamin C and folacin.

NUTRITIONAL INFORMATION Calories 182, Calories from Fat 17%, Fat 3 g, Saturated Fat 1 g, Cholesterol 48 mg, Sodium 298 mg, Total Carbohydrate 19 g, Dietary Fiber 2 g, Total Sugars 3 g, Protein 19 g

DIABETIC EXCHANGES 1 starch, 1 vegetable, 2 1/2 lean meat

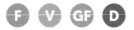

CREAMED DOUBLE POTATOES

Try this creamy, delicious mashed sweet and white potatoes combination that's easy to tolerate while getting valuable nutrition.

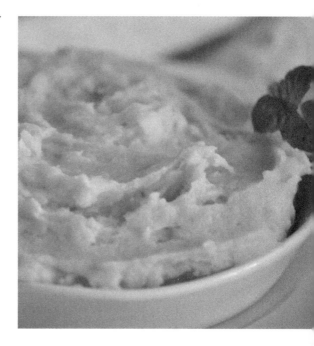

1 1/4 pounds baking potatoes, peeled and cut into chunks
1 1/4 pounds sweet potatoes, peeled and cut into chunks
1 tablespoon butter
2/3 cup skim milk
2 tablespoons honey
Salt and pepper to taste

1 In large pot, bring potatoes and enough water to cover to a boil. Boil 20–25 minutes or until potatoes are tender. Drain potatoes and transfer to a bowl.

2 Add remaining ingredients and mash until creamy.

MAKES 6 (2/3-cup) servings
PREP TIME 15 minutes
COOK TIME 25 minutes

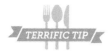

Softer and easy to swallow foods include cream soups, cheeses, mashed potatoes, pastas, yogurt, eggs, puddings, cooked cereals, ice cream, gravies, syrups, breakfast-type recipes, milkshakes, and nutritional liquid food supplements.

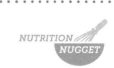

Baking potatoes are rich in vitamins B6, C, iron, magnesium, niacin, and potassium. Sweet potatoes provide vitamins A, B6, and C.

NUTRITIONAL INFORMATION Calories 292, Calories from Fat 9%, Fat 2 g, Saturated Fat 1 g, Cholesterol 6 mg, Sodium 86 mg, Total Carbohydrate 43 g, Dietary Fiber 5 g, Total Sugars 12 g, Protein 4 g

DIABETIC EXCHANGES 3 starch

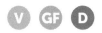

GLAZED CARROTS

Soft nutritous carrots tossed with a mild glaze give carrots a great flavor while being easy to eat.

1 (16-ounce) package baby carrots
1 tablespoon olive oil
2 tablespoons honey
1 teaspoon Dijon mustard
1/4 teaspoon ground ginger

1 In nonstick pot, steam carrots in water until very soft and tender. Drain cooking liquid.

2 In microwavable cup, microwave oil, honey, mustard, and ginger 20 seconds or until mixed. Toss with carrots.

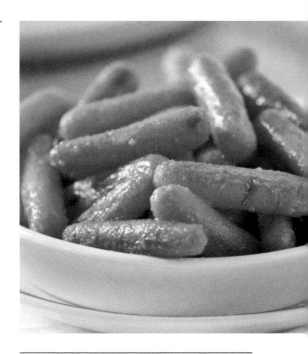

MAKES 6 (2/3-cup) servings
PREP TIME 5 minutes
COOK TIME 10 minutes

TERRIFIC TIP

Purchase baby carrots as less preparation and they cook quickly. Cut into small bite size pieces. Leave out the mustard if having severe issues.

. . . .

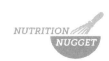
NUTRITION
NUGGET

Carrots are so well known for their extremely high antioxidant beta-carotene content they were named after it!

NUTRITIONAL INFORMATION Calories 73, Calories from fat 33%, Fat 3 g, Saturated Fat 0 g, Cholesterol 0 mg, Sodium 78 mg, Carbohydrate 12 g, Dietary Fiber 1 g, Total Sugars 10 g, Protein 1 g

DIABETIC EXCHANGES 1 vegetable, 1/2 other carbohydrate, 1/2 fat

SPINACH ARTICHOKE DIP

Here's my favorite spinach dip that explodes with flavors of creamy Brie and Parmesan. Just eat with a spoon or some soft crackers or bread.

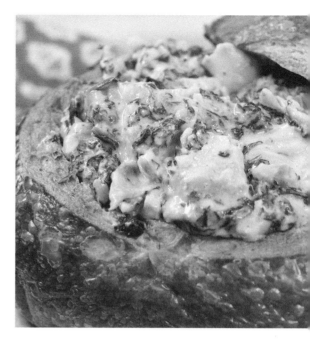

1 onion, finely chopped
1/3 cup all-purpose flour
2 cups skim milk
1 teaspoon minced garlic
2 (10-ounce) boxes frozen chopped spinach, thawed and drained
4 ounces Brie cheese, rind removed and cubed
1/3 cup grated Parmesan cheese
1 (14-ounce) can artichoke hearts, drained and finely chopped
Salt and pepper to taste

MAKES 20 (1/4-cup) servings

PREP TIME 15 minutes

1. In nonstick pot coated with nonstick cooking spray, sauté onion until tender. Stir in flour. Gradually add milk, stirring constantly, heating until bubbly and thickened.

2. Add garlic, spinach, Brie, and Parmesan cheese, stirring until cheese is melted. Stir in artichokes, and season to taste.

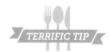

Keep in the refrigerator to pull out for a snack or serve as a side vegetable. Leave out the artichokes for a creamy spinach dip if your mouth is really sore.

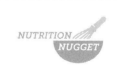

Between the spinach, milk and cheeses, this is a calcium-rich dish.

NUTRITIONAL INFORMATION Calories 54, Calories from fat 34%, Fat 2 g, Saturated Fat 1 g, Cholesterol 7 mg, Sodium 125 mg, Carbohydrate 5 g, Dietary Fiber 1 g, Total Sugars 2 g, Protein 4 g

DIABETIC EXCHANGES 1 vegetable, 1/2 fat

PREP TIME 5 minutes | COOK TIME 8 minutes

PREP TIME 10 minutes

MOCK MASHED POTATOES

When I served this dish to my family, not telling them it was cauliflower, they all raved about the flavor and went back for seconds. Your secret is safe with me!

- 1 medium head cauliflower, cut into florets
- 1/2 cup water
- 3 tablespoons grated Parmesan cheese
- 1/4 cup buttermilk
- 1/2 teaspoon minced garlic
- Salt and pepper to taste

1 In microwave-safe bowl, combine cauliflower and water, cover. Microwave 8 minutes or until tender.

2 Drain, place in blender or food processor with remaining ingredients. Blend until creamy, but do not overmix.

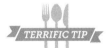

TERRIFIC TIP

Don't have buttermilk? Add 1 teaspoon lemon juice to 1/4 cup milk.

QUICK FLAN

A quick and simple light, melt-in-your mouth dessert or snack that feels and tastes good.

- 1 (3-ounce) package instant vanilla pudding and pie filling mix
- 1 3/4 cups skim milk
- 2 teaspoons vanilla

1 In bowl, whisk together pudding mix, milk and vanilla. Pour into 4 small ramekins.

2 Refrigerate 5–10 minutes or until set.

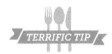

TERRIFIC TIP

Sometimes I like to use instant cream cheese pudding and pie filling mix.

· · · · · · · · · · · · · · · ·

DOC'S NOTE

This light dessert, along with other soft foods such as puddings, flavored gelatin, and cooked cereals are good to include in your diet when your throat is sore.

NUTRITIONAL INFORMATION Calories 59, Calories from fat 12%, Fat 1 g, Saturated Fat 1 g, Cholesterol 4 mg Sodium 117 mg, Carbohydrate 9 g, Dietary Fiber 4 g, Total Sugars 4 g, Protein 5 g

DIABETIC EXCHANGES 2 vegetable, 1/2 fat

NUTRITIONAL INFORMATION Calories 123, Calories from Fat 0%, Fat 0 g, Saturated Fat 0 g, Cholesterol 2 mg, Sodium 352 mg, Carbohydrates 25 g, Dietary Fiber 0 g, Total Sugars 25 g, Protein 4 g

DIABETIC EXCHANGES 1 1/2 carbohydrate, 1/2 fat-free milk

CREAM CHEESE BREAD PUDDING

Melt in your mouth bread pudding with a cream cheese topping makes this a light enjoyable dessert or snack that is easy to eat.

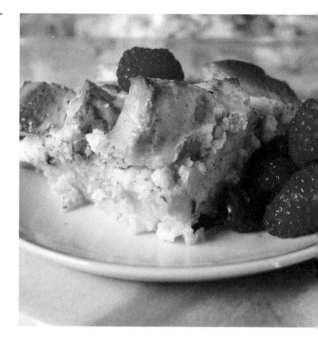

1 (16-ounce) loaf French bread
2 eggs, divided
4 egg whites, divided
1 cup sugar, divided
1 teaspoon vanilla extract
1 teaspoon butter flavoring
3 cups skim milk
1 teaspoon ground cinnamon
1 (8-ounce) package reduced-fat cream cheese

1 Preheat oven 350°F. Coat 13×9×2-inch baking dish with nonstick cooking spray.

2 Cut French bread into 1-inch squares. Place bread in prepared dish.

3 In large bowl, lightly beat together 1 egg and 3 egg whites. Add 1/2 cup sugar, vanilla, butter flavoring; mix well. Slowly add milk to egg mixture, mixing well. Pour over bread squares. Sprinkle mixture with cinnamon.

4 In mixing bowl, beat cream cheese with remaining 1/2 cup sugar. Add remaining egg and egg white, blending until smooth. Spread mixture evenly over soaked bread.

5 Bake, uncovered, 45 minutes or until firm. Let cool slightly before serving.

MAKES 16 servings
PREP TIME 15 minutes
COOK TIME 45 minutes

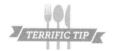
TERRIFIC TIP

When mouth and throat are sore, avoid tart, acidic, or salty foods and drinks such as citrus fruit juices (grapefruit, orange, lime), pickled and vinegary foods and tomato-based foods.

· · · · · · · · · · · · · · · · ·

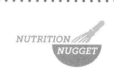
NUTRITION NUGGET

Depending on how you feel, you can add fruit to the bread pudding.

NUTRITIONAL INFORMATION Calories 197, Calories from Fat 19%, Fat 4 g, Saturated Fat 2 g, Cholesterol 34 mg, Sodium 248 mg, Carbohydrates 31 g, Dietary Fiber 1 g, Total Sugars 16 g, Protein 8 g

DIABETIC EXCHANGES 1 starch, 1 other carbohydrate, 1/2 lean meat

V **D**

PISTACHIO TIRAMISU WITH CHOCOLATE SAUCE

Whip up this effortlessly light soothing treat with layers of pistachio pudding, whipped topping and lady fingers drizzled with chocolate sauce.

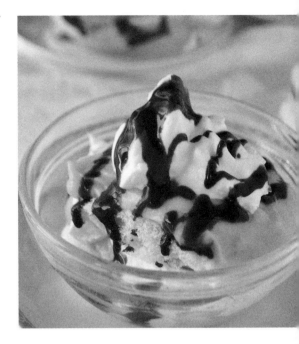

1 (4-serving) package instant sugar-free pistachio pudding and pie filling mix
1 3/4 cups skim milk
16 lady fingers or angel food cake slices
16 tablespoons fat-free frozen whipped topping, thawed
4 teaspoons chocolate syrup

1 In bowl, beat pudding mix with milk until thickens; set aside several minutes.

2 In each of four small serving bowls, layer 2 lady fingers, 1/4 cup pistachio pudding and 2 tablespoons whipped topping. Repeat layers ending with whipped topping. Drizzle each with 1 teaspoon chocolate syrup. Refrigerate.

MAKES 4 servings
PREP TIME 15 minutes

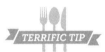
TERRIFIC TIP

You can always substitute different flavored puddings and leave off the chocolate sauce, if desired.

· · · · · · · · · · · · · · · · ·

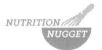
NUTRITION
NUGGET

By choosing low-fat dairy products you are actually getting more calcium, since the fat replaces the calcium in whole milk and cheeses.

NUTRITIONAL INFORMATION Calories 206, Calories from Fat 4%, Fat 1 g, Saturated Fat 0 g, Cholesterol 26 mg, Sodium 331 mg, Carbohydrates 41 g, Dietary Fiber 0 g, Total Sugars 23 g, Protein 5 g

DIABETIC EXCHANGES 2 1/2 other carbohydrate

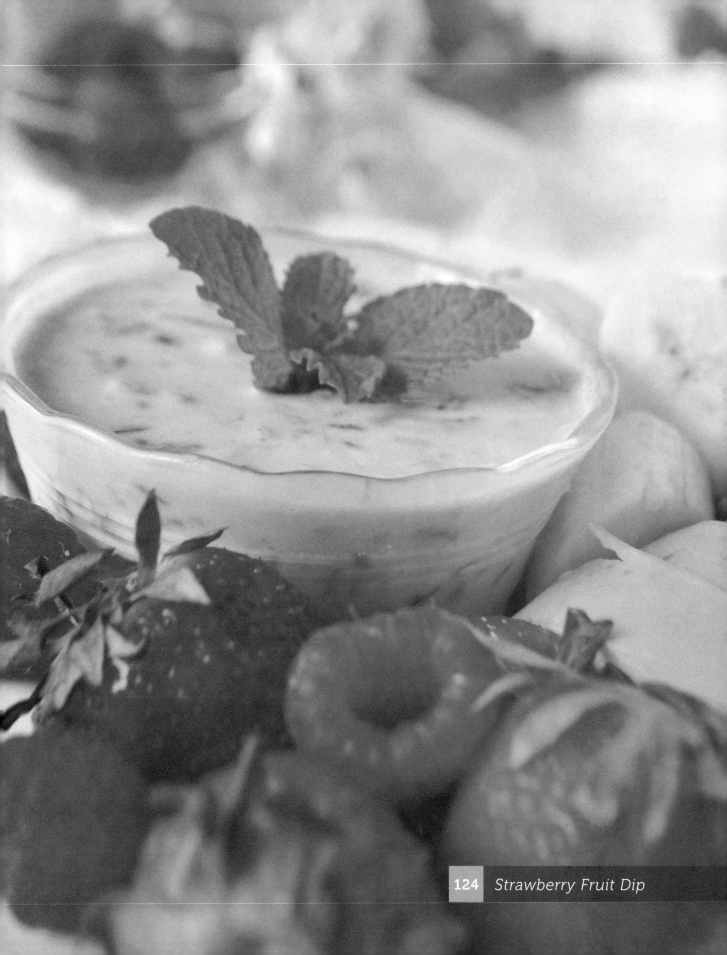

124 Strawberry Fruit Dip

HIGH CALORIE–HIGH PROTEIN

Recipes to improve immunity and healing, and help fight fatigue, weight loss and decrease of appetite that include increased calories and a good source of protein.

. . . .

Is weight loss a problem during treatment?

Can your appetite change during the day?

When I don't have an appetite, do I have to eat three large meals per day? If not, what should I do?

Why do I need more protein in my diet?

What are some good sources of protein?

· ·

Patients should try to avoid weight loss. Weight loss can be a serious problem for patients undergoing chemotherapy and/or radiation therapy. It has been proven that cancer patients who maintain their weight and maintain a good nutritional state tend to have fewer complications from chemotherapy, radiation therapy or surgery. These patients tend to have shorter hospital stays, reduced illness, fewer infections, have less of a down time and tend to better maintain strength and a sense of well-being.

It is very common for the appetite to decrease as the day progresses. If this occurs, make breakfast your big meal. If you crave or feel you can tolerate a steak and baked potato for breakfast, go for it!

Eating small meals throughout the day is very acceptable. Try eating small, frequent meals and snacks every one to two hours. Keep high-protein, high-calorie snacks and foods handy to eat when you are hungry. If solid foods don't appeal to you, try drinking liquids whenever possible. On the other hand, limit liquids with meals (unless needed to help swallow or for dry mouth) to keep from feeling full early. Avoid food smells when cooking as it can upset the appetite.

There are times that people with cancer need more protein. Protein helps to ensure growth, to repair body tissue, and to maintain a healthy immune system. Without enough protein, the body can take longer to recover from illness and you can have a lower resistance to infection. Following surgery, chemotherapy, and radiation therapy, additional protein is usually needed to heal tissues and to help prevent infection.

Good sources of protein include lean meat, fish, poultry, dairy products, nuts, dried beans, peas and lentils, and soy foods. Fortified milk is a great way to add protein to recipes.

TIPS FOR MORE CALORIES AND PROTEIN

- Keep snacks handy to have available all the time.

- Quick and easy snacks include: cheese and crackers, muffins, ice cream, peanut butter, dried fruit, and pudding are good possibilities.

- Take a portable snack with you when you go out, such as peanut butter crackers or small boxes of raisins.

- Even if you don't feel like eating solid foods, try to drink liquids during the day. Juice, soup, and other fluids give you important calories and nutrients. Milk-based drinks also provide protein.

- For extra protein in dishes, consider adding a little nonfat instant dry milk to scrambled eggs, soup, cereal, sauces, and gravies.

- Use instant breakfast powder in milk drinks, desserts, and ice cream.

- Try hard-cooked eggs, peanut butter, cheese, ice cream, granola bars, nutritional supplements, puddings, chips, crackers, and pretzels.

FOODS THAT PROVIDE 7 GRAMS OF PROTEIN PER SERVING

- 1 cup legumes
- 1–2 ounces nuts or seeds
- 1 cup cottage cheese
- 2 tablespoons peanut butter
- 1 ounce cheese
- 1 cup cooked wild rice
- 7 ounces milk or yogurt
- 1 cup tofu
- 2 tablespoons chicken breast
- 1 oz ground beef
- 2.5 ounces tempeh

HOW TO ADD PROTEIN AND/OR CALORIES TO YOUR DIET

Cheese
- Melt on soups, sandwiches, breads, muffins, omelets, casseroles, tortillas or any meat, chicken or fish.

Cottage cheese/ricotta/cream cheese
- Add to casseroles, spaghetti, and pasta.
- Use as stuffing for crepes, pasta shells, or manicotti.
- Add to omelets, scrambled eggs, and pancake batter.
- Spread cream cheese on bread, muffins, fruit and crackers.

Sour cream or yogurt
- Add to cream soups, baked potatoes, macaroni and cheese, vegetables, sauces, salad dressings, stews, baked meat, and fish.
- Use as a topping for cakes, fruit, gelatin desserts, breads, and muffins.
- Use as a dip for fresh fruits and vegetables.
- For dessert, scoop on fresh fruit, add brown sugar, and refrigerate until cold before eating.

Eggs
- Add chopped hard-boiled eggs to salads, vegetable dishes, and casseroles.
- Add extra eggs or egg whites to pancakes and French toast batter.
- Add extra eggs or egg whites to scrambled eggs and omelets.
- Add extra eggs or egg whites to custards and puddings.

Milk
- Use milk instead of water for liquid when cooking.
- Use in preparing hot cereal, soups, hot chocolate, and puddings.
- Use to make cream sauces for vegetables and other recipes.

Nonfat instant dry milk

- Add to milk and milk drinks.

- Use in casseroles, sauces, cream soups, mashed potatoes, custards and milk-based desserts.

Ice cream, yogurt and frozen yogurt

- Add to carbonated beverages, creating ice cream floats.

- Add to milk drinks like milk shakes.

- Serve ice cream or yogurt with cake, cookies, graham crackers or any dessert.

- Make breakfast drinks with fruit and bananas.

- Choose Greek yogurt when possible as it provides less sugar and more protein.

Soy

- Add tofu to shakes and dips.

- Snack on edamame or add to vegetable dishes, salads, and main dishes.

Peanut butter

- Spread on sandwiches, crackers, muffins, pancakes, fruit, and celery.

- Use as a dip for raw vegetables.

- Blend with milk drinks.

- Swirl with ice cream and frozen yogurt.

Meat and fish

- Add chopped cooked meat or fish to salads, casseroles, soups, and sauces.

- Use in omelets, quiches, sandwich filling, dressings and stuffings.

- Add to baked potato.

- When cooking meat, add a glaze or sauce.

Beans/legumes

- Add to soups, casseroles, pastas, and main dishes.

Nuts, seeds and wheat germ

- Add to casseroles, breads, muffins, pancakes, cookies, and waffles.

- Sprinkle on fruit, cereal, ice cream, vegetables, salads, and desserts.

- Roll fruit in nuts.

HOW TO INCREASE CALORIES:

Salad dressings and mayonnaise

- Spread on sandwiches.

- Combine with meat, fish, and egg or vegetable salads.

- Use in sauces and gelatin dishes.

Granola

- Use in cookie, muffin, and bread batters.

- Sprinkle on vegetables, yogurt, ice cream, pudding, custard, and fruit.

- Layer with fruits and bake.

- Mix with dry fruits and nuts for a snack.

- Substitute for bread or rice in pudding recipes.

Dried fruit

- Try cooking dried fruits for breakfast, snack or dessert.

- Add to muffins, cookies, breads, cakes, rice and grain dishes, cereals, puddings.

- Bake in pies and turnovers.

- Combine with cooked vegetables, such as carrots, sweet potatoes, yams, acorn squash and butternut squash.

- Combine with nuts or granola for snacks.

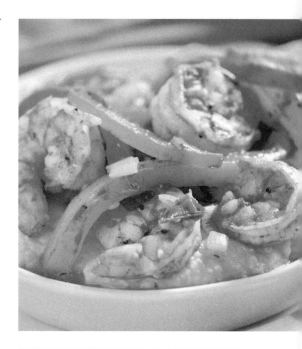

F **GF**

SHRIMP AND PEPPERS WITH CHEESE GRITS

Shrimp with vibrant peppers in a light flavorsome sauce served over creamy cheesy grits makes a great meal any time of the day.

3 assorted bell peppers, (red, green, yellow) cored and chopped
1 cup chopped Roma tomatoes
1 1/2 pounds medium peeled shrimp
1/2 cup chopped green onions
2 cups skim milk
1 1/2 cups water
1 cup quick grits
1 1/2 cups shredded reduced-fat sharp Cheddar cheese
1 tablespoon Worcestershire sauce

1 In large nonstick skillet coated with nonstick cooking spray, sauté bell peppers, tomatoes, and shrimp, cooking until shrimp are done, about 7 minutes. Add green onions.

2 Meanwhile, in nonstick pot bring milk and water to boil. Stir in grits. Return to boil, reduce heat, cover and cook about 5 minutes or until thickened, stirring occasionally. Stir in cheese and Worcestershire sauce. Serve shrimp over cheese grits.

MAKES 6 (3/4-cup) servings of shrimp mixture with grits

PREP TIME 15 minutes

COOK TIME 15 minutes

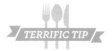

You can use less peppers for just a shrimp and cheese grits dish. Also, Louisiana crawfish (a good protein source) may be substituted for shrimp.

· · · · · · · · · · · · · · · · ·

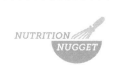

Reduced-fat dairy products actually give you more calcium, since the fat replaces the calcium in whole milk and cheese.

NUTRITIONAL INFORMATION Calories 301, Calories from fat 19%, Fat 6 g, Saturated Fat 3 g, Cholesterol 158 mg, Sodium 496 mg Carbohydrate 32 g, Dietary Fiber 2 g, Total Sugars 8 g, Protein 28 g

DIABETIC EXCHANGES 2 starch, 1 vegetable, 3 lean meat

SALMON AND ARTICHOKE PASTA SALAD

Fresh salmon is worth the extra effort, but to save time, you can substitute canned red salmon or tuna, or use leftover salmon.

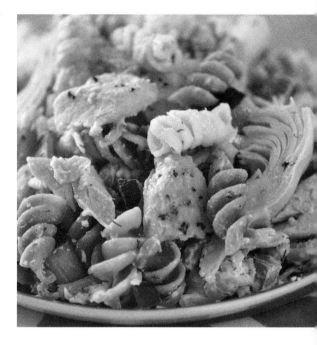

1 pound fresh salmon fillet
Salt and pepper to taste
1 (8-ounce) package rotini (spiral) pasta
1/3 cup light mayonnaise
1/2 cup nonfat plain yogurt
1/2 teaspoon sugar
2 teaspoons dried dill weed leaves
1/2 teaspoon white pepper
1 cup diced celery
1/2 cup chopped red onion
1 (14-ounce) can artichoke hearts, drained
  and quartered

1. Preheat oven 325°F. Line baking pan with foil and coat with nonstick cooking spray.

2. Season salmon and bake 15 minutes, or pan-fry, until salmon is done and flakes easily. Cool and remove skin, flake into chunks.

3. Cook pasta according to package directions. Drain, rinse, set aside.

4. In small bowl, mix mayonnaise, yogurt, sugar, dill weed, and pepper; set aside. In large bowl, mix together celery, red onion, artichokes, pasta, and mayonnaise mixture. Carefully add flaked salmon, tossing gently. Refrigerate until serving.

MAKES 6 (1 1/3-cup) servings
PREP TIME 10 minutes
COOK TIME 20 minutes

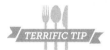

Fresh herbs may be substituted for dried herbs at a ratio of 3:1. In other words, 1 teaspoon of a dried herb equals 1 tablespoon fresh.

Not only is salmon rich in omega-3 fatty acids, it is also an excellent source of bone maintaining vitamin D and selenium—helping prevent oxidative stress and inflammation.

NUTRITIONAL INFORMATION Calories 307, Calories from Fat 21%, Fat 7 g, Saturated Fat 1 g, Cholesterol 40 mg, Sodium 327 mg, Carbohydrates 36 g, Dietary Fiber 2 g, Total Sugars 5 g, Protein 23 g

DIABETIC EXCHANGES 2 starch, 1 vegetable, 2 lean meat

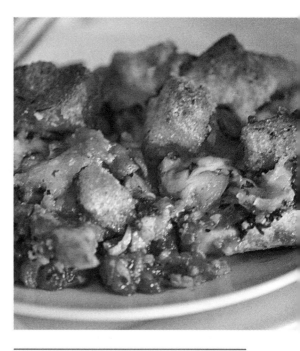

CHICKEN PARMESAN ONE-DISH

An amazing tasting 6-ingredient one-dish time-saver version with chicken, marinara, basil, cheese and croutons. Serve with pasta.

2 pounds thin boneless, skinless chicken breast cutlets
Salt and pepper to taste
1 tablespoon minced garlic
2 cups healthy marinara sauce
1 tablespoon dried basil leaves
1 1/2 cups shredded part-skim mozzarella cheese, divided
1 (5-ounce) package Caesar or garlic croutons

1 Preheat oven 350°F. Coat 3-quart baking dish with nonstick cooking spray.

2 Season chicken and mix with garlic in prepared baking dish. Cover with marinara and sprinkle with basil.

3 Sprinkle with half the mozzarella, all the croutons and top with remaining mozzarella. Bake 40–50 minutes or until chicken is tender.

MAKES 8 servings (about 1-cup each)
PREP TIME 15 minutes
COOK TIME 50 minutes

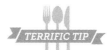

TERRIFIC TIP

Thin chicken breasts in the grocery are also called chicken cutlets. If croutons start getting too brown, cover with foil at the end of cooking.

· · · · · · · · · · · · · · · · ·

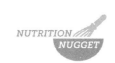

NUTRITION NUGGET

Look for jars of 'healthy' marina sauce that offer lower sodium and lower sugar.

NUTRITIONAL INFORMATION Calories 320, Calories from Fat 34%, Fat 12 g, Saturated Fat 3 g, Cholesterol 84 mg, Sodium 678 mg, Carbohydrates 18 g, Dietary Fiber 2 g, Total Sugars 8 g, Protein 33 g

DIABETIC EXCHANGES 1 starch, 4 lean meat

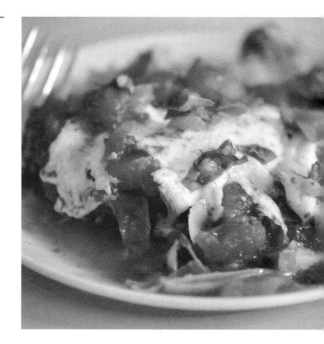

GF

CAPRESE CHICKEN BAKE

Tomatoes, basil and mozzarella cook with chicken for a superb moist, full flavored chicken bake.

3 cups chopped Roma tomatoes
1 cup chopped onion
1 (14-ounce) can artichoke hearts quartered, drained
1 tablespoon minced garlic
2 tablespoons olive oil
3 tablespoons balsamic vinegar
Salt and pepper to taste
1 1/2 pounds boneless, skinless thin chicken breasts
  or tenders
2 ounces fresh mozzarella, thinly sliced
1/4 cup fresh chopped basil leaves

1 Preheat oven 375°F. In large oblong baking dish, combine tomatoes, onion, artichoke hearts, garlic, olive oil, balsamic vinegar and season to taste.

2 Add chicken breasts and toss together spreading out in prepared baking dish. Bake 30–40 minutes or until chicken is tender.

3 Remove from oven and top chicken breasts with mozzarella. Return to oven 5 minutes or until cheese is melted. Sprinkle with basil.

MAKES 4 servings
PREP TIME 15 minutes
COOK TIME 40 minutes

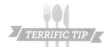
TERRIFIC TIP

If you like more cheese, you can add extra slices. Dried basil and grated part-skim mozzarella cheese may be used instead of fresh mozzarella.

. . . .

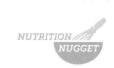
NUTRITION NUGGET

Artichokes are a naturally low-sodium, fat-free, low-calorie food, rich in healthy antioxidants and phytonutrients.

NUTRITIONAL INFORMATION Calories 384, Calories from Fat 35%, Fat 15 g, Saturated Fat 3 g, Cholesterol 123 mg, Sodium 517 mg, Carbohydrates 17 g, Dietary Fiber 3 g, Total Sugars 9 g, Protein 45 g

DIABETIC EXCHANGES 3 vegetable, 5 lean meat

(F) (GF)

CHICKEN AND BLACK BEAN ENCHILADAS

These delicious enchiladas pack tons of flavor and also freeze well to pull out for meals on days you don't feel like cooking—freeze before baking.

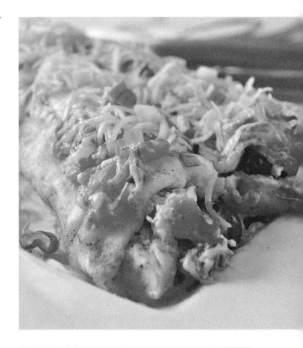

1 1/4 pounds skinless, boneless chicken breasts, cut into chunks or strips
1/2 teaspoon minced garlic
1 1/2 cups salsa, divided
1 (15-ounce) can black beans, rinsed and drained
1 red or green bell pepper, cored and chopped
1 teaspoon ground cumin
1 bunch green onions, chopped
12 (6–8-inch) flour tortillas (use corn for gluten-free)
6 ounces reduced-fat Mexican-blend cheese, shredded

MAKES 12 enchiladas (2 per serving)
PREP TIME 20 minutes
COOK TIME 15 minutes

1 Preheat oven 350°F. Coat 13×9×2-inch baking dish with nonstick cooking spray.

2 In nonstick skillet coated with nonstick cooking spray, sauté chicken and garlic until chicken is almost done, 5-7 minutes.

3 Stir in 1/2 cup salsa, beans, bell pepper, and cumin. Cook on low heat until thickened, about 5 minutes, stirring occasionally, or until chicken is done. Stir in green onions.

4 Divide chicken-bean mixture among 12 tortillas, placing mixture down center of each tortilla. Top with 1 tablespoon shredded cheese. Roll up and place seam-side down in prepared dish.

5 Spoon remaining 1 cup salsa evenly over enchiladas. Top with remaining cheese. Bake 15 minutes, or until thoroughly heated and cheese melted.

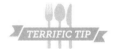
TERRIFIC TIP

Take a short cut and subsitute skinless rotesserie chicken for chicken breasts. You can also serve one enchilada per person depending on the meal.

· · · · · · · · · · · · · · · · · ·

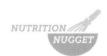
NUTRITION
NUGGET

Move over orange juice, 1 cup bell pepper provides 200% of your daily recommendation of vitamin C.

NUTRITIONAL INFORMATION Calories 454, Calories from Fat 17%, Fat 8 g, Saturated Fat 4 g, Cholesterol 76 mg, Sodium 1267 mg, Carbohydrates 54 g, Dietary Fiber 6 g, Total Sugars 4 g, Protein 36 g

DIABETIC EXCHANGES 3 starch, 1 vegetable, 4 lean meat

F **GF** **D**

CUBAN PORK AND BLACK BEANS

Pork tenderloins cooked with black beans and southwestern seasoning make this an ideal recipe for a slow cooker. Serve with yellow rice.

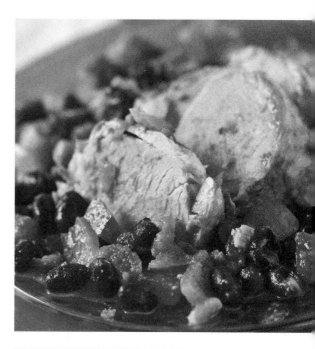

2 (1-pound) pork tenderloins
Garlic powder
2 onions, chopped
1 (15-ounce) can black bean soup
1 (15-ounce) can black beans, rinsed and drained
1 (10-ounce) can tomatoes and green chilies
1 tablespoon chopped jalapeños
2 tablespoons ground cumin
2 tablespoons lime juice

1 Season pork tenderloins heavily with garlic powder.

2 In 3 1/2–6-quart slow cooker combine all ingredients.

3 Cook on LOW 6–8 hours or until pork tenderloin is tender.

MAKES 10 servings
PREP TIME 10 minutes
COOK TIME 6–8 hours in slow cooker

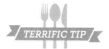
TERRIFIC TIP

Don't peek! If you leave the top off the slow cooker, you can lose up to 20 degrees of cooking heat in as little as 2 minutes.

· · · · · · · · · · · · · · · ·

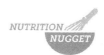
NUTRITION
NUGGET

A nutritional gem, beans provide an excellent source of fiber and folate, helping with digestive health and weight maintenance.

NUTRITIONAL INFORMATION Calories 245, Calories from Fat 23%, Fat 6 g, Saturated Fat 2 g, Cholesterol 76 mg, Sodium 527 mg, Carbohydrates 17 g, Dietary Fiber 5 g, Total Sugars 5 g, Protein 29 g

DIABETIC EXCHANGES 1 starch, 1 vegetable, 4 lean meat

F **D**

TROUT WITH PECANS AND DIJON SAUCE

Liven up broiled fish with this simple, scrumptious sauce and toasted pecans for a mild, delicious fish recipe.

6 (4-ounce) trout fillets
Salt and pepper to taste
1/2 cup Italian bread crumbs
1/4 cup nonfat plain yogurt
2 teaspoons Dijon mustard
1 tablespoon lemon juice
3 tablespoons chopped pecans, toasted
1/2 cup chopped green onions

1 Preheat broiler.

2 Season fish to taste and arrange in oblong baking dish coated with nonstick cooking spray. Top fish evenly with bread crumbs. Cook under broiler 5–7 minutes, or until fish flakes easily when tested with fork.

3 Meanwhile, in small bowl, combine yogurt, mustard, and lemon juice. Spoon 1 tablespoon sauce over each fish fillet and sprinkle with pecans and green onions.

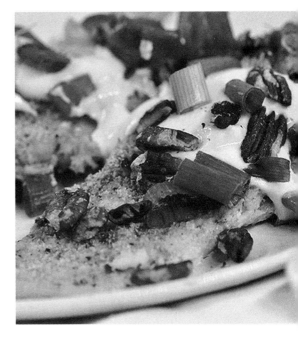

MAKES 6 servings
PREP TIME 10 minutes
COOK TIME 7 minutes

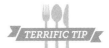
TERRIFIC TIP

To test fish for doneness, prod it with a fork at its thickest point. Properly cooked fish is opaque, has milky white juices and just begins to flake easily. Don't overcook or it will be dry.

· · · · · · · · · · · · · · · · · ·

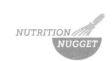
NUTRITION NUGGET

Trout is a mild fish rich in amino acids—precursors to protein, important building blocks for healing and tissue repair.

NUTRITIONAL INFORMATION Calories 206, Calories from Fat 32%, Fat 7 g, Saturated Fat 1 g, Cholesterol 67 mg, Sodium 246 mg, Carbohydrates 8 g, Dietary Fiber 1 g, Total Sugars 1 g, Protein 26 g

DIABETIC EXCHANGES 3 lean meat, 1/2 starch

SALMON AND KALE PASTA

Simple ingredients, easy preparation and a sensational salmon dish. Roast salmon in the oven, cook pasta and stir fry kale and tomatoes to toss together.

1 pound skinless salmon fillet
Salt and pepper
2 tablespoons lemon juice, divided
8 ounces rotini pasta
2 tablespoons olive oil
3 cups packed fresh baby kale
1 cup chopped tomatoes
1 teaspoon minced garlic
1/4 cup chopped green onion stems
Grated Parmesan cheese, optional

1. Preheat oven to 425°F. Coat baking pan with foil and nonstick cooking spray.

2. Season salmon to taste. Drizzle with 1 tablespoon lemon juice. Roast salmon 12 minutes or until flakes with fork. Cut into chunks.

3. Meanwhile, cook pasta according to directions. Drain; set aside.

4. In large nonstick skillet, heat olive oil and quickly cook kale, tomatoes and garlic until kale is slightly wilted, about 3 minutes. Add remaining tablespoon lemon juice. Carefully stir in pasta and salmon, cooking until heated through. Top with green onions and grated Parmesan cheese, if desired.

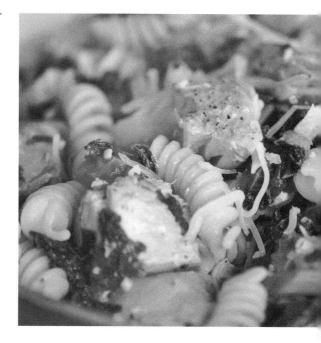

MAKES 7 (1-cup) servings
PREP TIME 15 minutes
COOK TIME 20 minutes

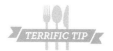
TERRIFIC TIP

You can substitute baby spinach for the kale.

· · · · · · · · · · · · · · · ·

DOC'S NOTE

At least two servings of fish (fatty fish preferred) per week for heart health is the recommended intake by the American Heart Association.

NUTRITIONAL INFORMATION Calories 260, Calories from Fat 27%, Fat 8 g, Saturated Fat 1 g, Cholesterol 30 mg, Sodium 66 mg, Carbohydrates 28 g, Dietary Fiber 2 g, Total Sugars 2 g, Protein 19 g

DIABETIC EXCHANGES 1 1/2 starch, 1 vegetable, 2 lean meat

F D

TUNA WITH BROCCOLI AND WHITE BEAN PASTA

Slices of seared tuna top a mixture of broccoli, white beans and pasta in a light broth sauce.

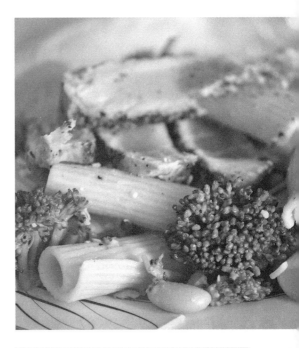

12 ounces rigatoni or tubular pasta
2 tablespoons olive oil
4 cups broccoli florets
1 teaspoon minced garlic
2 cups fat-free chicken broth
1 (16-ounce) can cannelloni beans, drained and rinsed
1 1/2 pounds tuna filets
Salt and pepper taste
1/4 cup grated Parmesan cheese

1 Prepare pasta according to package directions. Drain, set aside.

2 In large nonstick skillet, heat olive oil over medium heat, stir-fry broccoli and garlic about 5 minutes until broccoli is crisp tender. Add chicken broth and cannelloni beans. Bring to boil and add pasta, toss together.

3 Meanwhile, season tuna to taste. In heated nonstick skillet coated with nonstick cooking spray, sear tuna on both sides, 3–5 minutes, depending on doneness. Slice tuna. Sprinkle Parmesan cheese over pasta and serve with sliced tuna.

MAKES 6 (1 2/3 cups) servings of pasta with 4 ounces sliced tuna

PREP TIME 15 minutes

COOK TIME 20 minutes

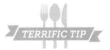

The tuna may be omitted for a flavorful vegetarian pasta dish.

· · · · · · · · · · · · · · · ·

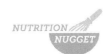

Tuna is a great source of protein and omega 3 fatty acids and the beans and cheese are added protein.

NUTRITIONAL INFORMATION Calories 457, Calories from Fat 16%, Fat 8 g, Saturated Fat 2 g, Cholesterol 56 mg, Sodium 541 mg, Carbohydrates 56 g, Dietary Fiber 6 g, Total Sugars 2 g, Protein 38 g

DIABETIC EXCHANGES 3 1/2 starch, 1 vegetable, 4 lean meat

MARINATED FLANK STEAK

Marinade is the key to adding flavor to flank steak. For a terrific quick meal, this is a go-to marinade. Flat iron or skirt steak may also be used.

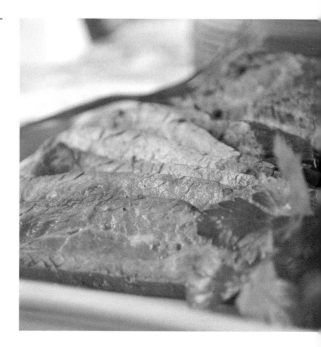

- 3 tablespoons low-sodium soy sauce
- 3 tablespoons honey
- 1 1/2 teaspoons garlic powder
- 1/2 teaspoon ground ginger or 1 1/2 teaspoons chopped fresh ginger
- 1 green onion, chopped
- 2 pounds flank steak, trimmed of excess fat

1 In large plastic bag or glass dish, mix together all ingredients except flank steak. Add flank steak, refrigerate, and marinate 2 hours or time permitted, turning occasionally.

2 Discard marinade. Grill flank steak over hot fire until cooked rare to medium rare, 4-7 minutes on each side. May be broiled in oven. Serve rare, let sit 5 minutes before slicing. Cut diagonally across grain into thin slices.

MAKES 6 (4-ounce) servings

PREP TIME 5 minutes + time to marinate

COOK TIME 15 minutes

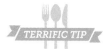

Make this simple marinade instead of buying it, there will be less sodium.

· · · · · · · · · · · · · · · · · ·

Garlic in foods can add more than flavor—as garlic is high in antioxidant content, helping to boost your immune system easing inflammation.

NUTRITIONAL INFORMATION Calories 219, Calories from Fat 37%, Fat 9 g, Saturated Fat 4 g, Cholesterol 64 mg, Sodium 250 mg, Carbohydrates 1 g, Dietary Fiber 0 g, Total Sugars 1 g, Protein 32 g

DIABETIC EXCHANGES 4 lean meat

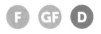

QUICK CHILI

Meat, salsa, corn, beef broth and beans are the foundation for this incredible quick and popular chili.

2 pounds ground sirloin
1 teaspoon minced garlic
1 tablespoon chili powder
1 teaspoon ground cumin
1 (16-ounce) jar salsa
1 (16-ounce) package frozen corn
2 (14 1/2-ounce) cans seasoned low-sodium
  fat-free beef broth
1 (15-ounce) can pinto beans, rinsed and drained

1 In large nonstick pot, cook meat and garlic until done; drain excess fat. Add remaining ingredients.

2 Bring mixture to boil, reduce heat and cook 15 minutes.

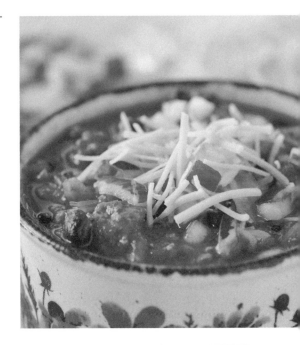

MAKES 8 (1-cup) servings
PREP TIME 15 minutes
COOK TIME 15 minutes

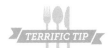
TERRIFIC TIP

Keep canned beans on hand for an easy, pantry friendly protein source—rinse and drain to cut sodium by up to 40%.

. . . .

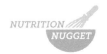
NUTRITION NUGGET

This dish is full of great sources of protein, such as beef and beans. Other good protein sources include fish, poultry, dairy products, nuts, dried beans, lentils and soy foods.

NUTRITIONAL INFORMATION Calories 264, Calories from Fat 21%, Fat 6 g, Saturated Fat 2 g, Cholesterol 62 mg, Sodium 464 mg, Carbohydrates 25 g, Dietary Fiber 5 g, Total Sugars 4 g, Protein 30 g

DIABETIC EXCHANGES 1 1/2 starch, 1 vegetable, 3 lean meat

EASY MEAT SAUCE

By using a jar of marinara with fresh vegetables, you get an easy and amazing homemade sauce. Serve with your favorite pasta.

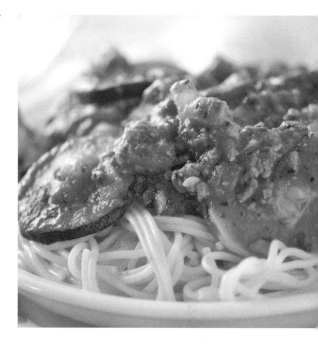

1 large onion, chopped
1 medium yellow squash, thinly sliced
1 medium zucchini, thinly sliced
2 pounds ground sirloin
1 tablespoon minced garlic
1 (24-ounce) jar marinara sauce
1 tablespoon dried basil leaves
1 tablespoon dried oregano leaves
Pinch sugar
Salt and pepper to taste

1. In large nonstick skillet coated with nonstick cooking spray, sauté onion, squash, and zucchini about 5 minutes. Add meat and garlic and cook over medium heat until meat is done and vegetables are tender, 5–7 minutes. Drain excess grease.

2. Add marinara, basil, oregano and sugar. Bring to boil, stirring constantly. Reduce heat, and simmer, uncovered, 20 minutes. Season to taste.

MAKES 8 (1-cup) servings
PREP TIME 15 minutes
COOK TIME 30–35 minutes

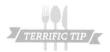
TERRIFIC TIP

Meat sauce freezes great so freeze in individual zip-top freezer bags to pull out for meals.

· · · · · · · · · · · · · · · · ·

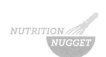
NUTRITION
NUGGET

Ensure you are choosing the leanest cuts of meat by looking for those ending in "loin" or "round."

NUTRITIONAL INFORMATION Calories 220, Calories from fat 31%, Fat 8 g, Saturated Fat 3 g, Cholesterol 62 mg Sodium 438 mg, Carbohydrate 12 g, Dietary Fiber 3 g, Total Sugars 3 g, Protein 27 g

DIABETIC EXCHANGES 2 vegetable, 3 lean meat

CABBAGE ROLL CASSEROLE

All the components of cabbage rolls combined into this scrumptious effortless casserole. The cabbage evaporates creating a moist great tasting casserole.

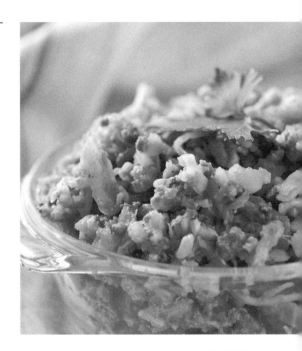

1 1/2 pounds ground sirloin
1 onion, chopped
1 teaspoon minced garlic
1/4 teaspoon pepper
3 cups instant brown rice
1 (16-ounce) bag cole slaw (shredded cabbage)
1 (24–26-ounce) jar healthy marinara sauce
1/4 cup light brown sugar

1 Preheat oven 350°F. Coat large oblong dish with nonstick baking spray.

2 In large nonstick skillet, cook meat, onion, and garlic until meat is done, about 8 minutes. Drain excess liquid. Add pepper and rice, mixing well. Spoon into prepared baking dish.

3 Top with cole slaw. In bowl, mix together marinara sauce and brown sugar. Pour sauce over cabbage.

4 Bake, covered, 1 hour and 15 minutes, or until cabbage is tender and rice is done.

MAKES 8 (1-cup) servings
PREP TIME 15 minutes
COOK TIME 1 hour and 25 minutes

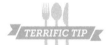
TERRIFIC TIP

Slow Cooker Directions: Follow directions in steps 2 and 3, but transfer ingredients to slow cooker rather than baking dish. Cover and cook on LOW 4-6 hours.

. . . .

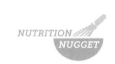
NUTRITION NUGGET

Filled with good for you nutrients such as fiber and calcium, cabbage is a veggie not to be overlooked.

NUTRITIONAL INFORMATION Calories 359, Calories from Fat 19%, Fat 8 g, Saturated Fat 2 g, Cholesterol 47 mg, Sodium 396 mg, Carbohydrates 48 g, Dietary Fiber 5 g, Total Sugars 16 g, Protein 23 g

DIABETIC EXCHANGES 3 starch, 1 vegetable, 2 1/2 lean meat

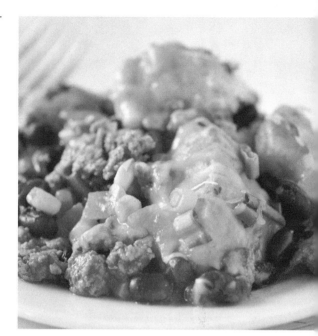

SIMPLE SOUTHWESTERN CASSEROLE

This zesty, meaty casserole with a biscuit surprise can be made in minutes! You'll be amazed at how extraordinarily tasty this simple combination is.

1 pound ground sirloin
1 onion, chopped
1 (10-ounce) can enchilada sauce
1 (8-ounce) can tomato sauce
1 (15-ounce) can black beans, rinsed and drained
1 cup frozen corn
1 (8-10 count) can reduced-fat refrigerator biscuits
1 cup shredded reduced-fat Mexican blend cheese
1/3 cup chopped green onions

1. Preheat oven 350°F. Coat 13×9×2-inch baking dish with nonstick cooking spray.

2. In large nonstick skillet, cook meat and onion until meat is done; drain excess fat. Add enchilada sauce, tomato sauce, black beans and corn, stirring well. Cut biscuits into fourths and stir into meat mixture.

3. Transfer to prepared pan. Bake 25 minutes. Remove from oven, sprinkle with cheese and green onions. Return to oven and bake 5–7 minutes more or until cheese is melted.

MAKES 9 (1-cup) servings
PREP TIME 10 minutes
COOK TIME 30–35 minutes

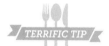
TERRIFIC TIP

Use kitchen scissors to make cutting biscuits easy. If you have trouble finding enchilada sauce, you can substitute salsa. Ground turkey may be substituted for the ground sirloin.

· · · · · · · · · · · · · · · · ·

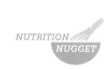
NUTRITION
NUGGET

Use full fat cheese and biscuits when trying to increase caloric intake.

NUTRITIONAL INFORMATION Calories 257, Calories from Fat 28%, Fat 8 g, Saturated Fat 4 g, Cholesterol 36 mg, Sodium 815 mg, Carbohydrates 27 g, Dietary Fiber 4 g, Total Sugars 5 g, Protein 20 g

DIABETIC EXCHANGES 1 1/2 starch, 1 vegetable, 2 lean meat

SNACKS + SMOOTHIES

Quick and easy recipes for small nutritious meals throughout the day:
as well as cool smoothing smoothies for effortless and odorless meals.

. . . .

Is snacking permissible?

Should I make snacks ahead of time?

Are smoothies a good snack?

. . . .

Snacking is not only permissible but strongly encouraged. It is often very hard to sit down for a full five-course meal, but easier to sit down to a thirty minute meal with two to three snacks in between. High calorie, low volume snacks are important to help you to maintain your weight. We will try to offer suggestions for snacks that can be made easily and with minimal effort.

Smoothies also make a good snack especially when your mouth is sore or you prefer odorless foods. A creamy cool smoothie can soothe the mouth and is an easy way to add nutrition. A quick smoothie is always a good way to sneak in extra fruit and veggies in your diet, combining frozen berries, spinach, Greek yogurt, nut butter and ice. Berries are rich in antioxidants, Greek yogurt is great source of calcium and protein while low in added sugar, and spinach is packed with calcium, iron and fiber—making it a nutrient rich light meal or snack. If frozen foods are too cold on your sore mouth, eliminate the ice and choose refrigerated or room temperature berries and foods to add to your smoothie.

SNACK FOOD IDEAS

- Applesauce
- Bread, muffins, and crackers
- Cereal
- Cheese
- Dips
- Eggs
- Fruit (fresh, canned, dried)
- Granola
- Hummus with pita bread
- Ice cream frozen yogurt, popsicles
- Juices
- Milk
- Milkshakes, instant breakfast drinks
- Nuts
- Peanut butter
- Pizza
- Popcorn
- Puddings and custards
- Sandwiches
- Smoothies
- Soups
- Vegetables (raw or cooked)
- Yogurt

F V

EASY CRANBERRY YAM BREAD

Get a quick start using biscuit baking mix, then add cream cheese for a rich flavor, naturally sweet yams to give the bread a natural sweetness, and cranberries for a burst of tartness.

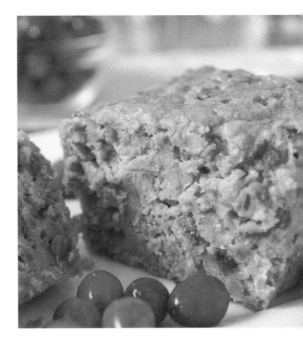

1 (8-ounce) package reduced-fat cream cheese
1 cup sugar
1 (15-ounce) can sweet potatoes, drained and mashed
2 eggs
1 1/2 cups biscuit baking mix
1 teaspoon ground cinnamon
1 cup dried cranberries or 1 cup chopped fresh
   cranberries

1 Preheat oven 350°F. Coat 9×5×3-inch loaf pan with nonstick cooking spray.

2 In large bowl, beat together cream cheese and sugar until light and fluffy. Beat in sweet potatoes and eggs. Stir in biscuit mix, cinnamon, and cranberries until just blended. Transfer to prepared pan.

3 Bake 45 minutes to an hour, or until toothpick inserted in center comes out clean. Cool in pan 15 minutes before serving.

MAKES 16 slices
PREP TIME 10 minutes
COOK TIME 45 minutes–1 hour

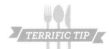

Fresh cranberries freeze for one year. Quick breads freeze well also.

· · · · · · · · · · · · · · · ·

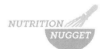

Cranberries provide a host of health benefits due to their high vitamin C and antioxidant properties, including tissue repair and growth, and urinary tract infection prevention.

NUTRITIONAL INFORMATION Calories 189, Calories from Fat 26%, Fat 6 g, Saturated Fat 3 g, Cholesterol 37 mg, Sodium 231 mg, Carbohydrates 31 g, Dietary Fiber 1 g, Total Sugars 19 g, Protein 4 g
DIABETIC EXCHANGES 1 1/2 starch, 1/2 fruit, 1 fat

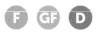

BANANA OATMEAL MUFFINS

You'll love this toss-in-the-food-processor, one bowl, moist, not-too-sweet banana muffin that's also gluten-free.

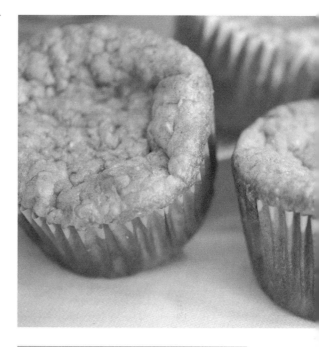

2 1/2 cups old-fashioned oatmeal
1 cup nonfat plain or vanilla Greek yogurt
2 eggs
1/2 cup light brown sugar
2 teaspoons baking powder
1 teaspoon baking soda
1 teaspoon vanilla extract
2 large ripe bananas

1 Preheat oven 350°F. Line muffin pans with papers and coat with nonstick cooking spray

2 Place oatmeal in food processor or blender and pulse about 10 seconds. Add remaining ingredients and process until mixture is smooth.

3 Divide batter among muffin papers. Bake 16-18 minutes, or until toothpick comes out clean. Let sit before removing from tins.

MAKES 18 muffins
PREP TIME 10 minutes
COOK TIME 18 minutes

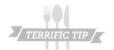

You can add your favorite nuts and dried fruit.

· · · · · · · · · · · · · · · · ·

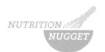

Greek yogurt is an excellent low-fat, low-sugar, high-protein substitute for plain yogurt or even sour cream.

NUTRITIONAL INFORMATION Calories 94, Calories from Fat 13%, Fat 1 g, Saturated Fat 0 g, Cholesterol 21 mg, Sodium 129 mg, Carbohydrates 17 g, Dietary Fiber 2 g, Total Sugars 9 g, Protein 4 g
DIABETIC EXCHANGES 1 starch

BLUEBERRY SURPRISE MUFFINS

Blueberries and, surprisingly, avocado—two of my favorites—make up this delicious moist muffin.

2 cups all-purpose flour
2 teaspoons baking powder
1/2 teaspoon baking soda
1/2 teaspoon ground cinnamon
1 ripe avocado, seeded and peeled (about 1/2–2/3 cup)
2/3 cup sugar
1 egg
1 1/2 teaspoons vanilla extract

1 cup nonfat plain Greek yogurt
2 cups fresh blueberries

Crumble Topping

1 tablespoon butter, melted
3 tablespoons all-purpose flour
2 tablespoons sugar
1/2-1 teaspoon vanilla extract

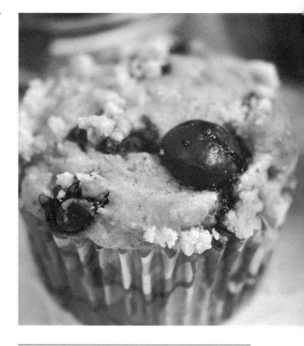

MAKES 18 muffins
PREP TIME 15 minutes
COOK TIME 30 minutes

1 Preheat oven 375°F. Line muffin tin with paper liners.

2 In medium bowl, stir together flour, baking powder, baking soda, and cinnamon; set aside.

3 In mixing bowl, beat avocado and sugar until smooth and well blended. Add egg, and continue beating until light. Add vanilla and yogurt, mixing until just combined.

4 Gradually add flour mixture, mixing until just combined. Gently fold in blueberries.

5 *For the Crumble Topping:* In small bowl, mix ingredients together with fork until crumbly.

6 Spoon batter into paper liners, and sprinkle with Crumble Topping. Bake 25–30 minutes, or until toothpick comes out clean.

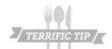

TERRIFIC TIP

Muffins freeze well to pull out for a snack whenever you want.

NUTRITION NUGGET

Blueberries, avocado and Greek yogurt provide a nutritional boost and make this a super-food muffin.

NUTRITIONAL INFORMATION Calories 130, Calories from Fat 16%, Fat 2 g, Saturated Fat 1 g, Cholesterol 12 mg, Sodium 95 mg, Carbohydrates 24 g, Dietary Fiber 1 g, Total Sugars 11 g, Protein 3 g

DIABETIC EXCHANGES 1 1/2 starch

HARVEST GRANOLA

Fantastic and versatile—you are in for a granola treat with all these fabulous seeds, berries, nuts, and spices.

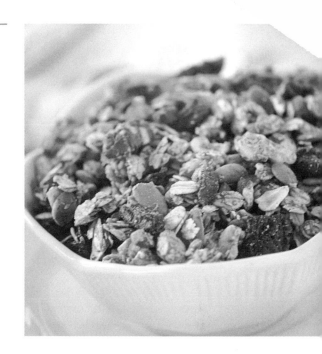

1/4 cup mashed sweet potatoes
2 tablespoons butter
2 tablespoons molasses
1/3 cup maple syrup
4 cups old-fashioned oatmeal
1/3 cup pumpkin seeds
1/2 cup dried cranberries
1/4 cup coarsely chopped pecans
1/3 cup coarsely chopped walnuts
1 teaspoon ground cinnamon
1/4 teaspoon ground cloves
Hearty dash salt

1 Preheat oven 300°F. Line baking pan with foil and coat with nonstick cooking spray.

2 In microwave-safe dish, combine sweet potatoes, butter, molasses and maple syrup. Microwave about 3 minutes or until bubbly.

3 In large bowl, combine remaining ingredients. Pour sweet potato mixture over oatmeal mixture, tossing until well mixed. Transfer to prepared pan and bake 35–40 minutes, stirring mixture about half way through. Cool.

MAKES 28 (1/4-cup) servings
PREP TIME 15 minutes
COOK TIME 40 minutes

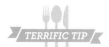
TERRIFIC TIP

You can adjust the different dried fruit, nuts and seeds to your preference. Use canned or leftover cooked sweet potatoes.

· · · · · · · · · · · · · · · · ·

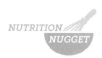
NUTRITION NUGGET

Great for breakfast, snack and to top yogurt—be sure to choose Greek yogurt for extra protein and low sugar.

NUTRITIONAL INFORMATION Calories 99, Calories from Fat 36%, Fat 4 g, Saturated Fat 1 g, Cholesterol 2 mg, Sodium 9 mg, Carbohydrates 14 g, Dietary Fiber 2 g, Total Sugars 5 g, Total Sugars 5 g, Protein 2 g
DIABETIC EXCHANGES 1 starch, 1/2 fat

_EAL MIX

Tasty _and terrific honey-peanut butter snack to keep on hand. It also helps stimulate you to drink fluids._

2 tablespoons honey
3 tablespoons peanut butter
3 cups cereal (assorted shredded wheat, oatmeal chex, corn bran chex)

1 Preheat oven 175°F. Line baking pan with foil coated with nonstick cooking spray.

2 In microwave-safe dish, microwave honey and peanut butter about 20 seconds or until smooth. Toss with cereal, coating well. Spread on prepared baking pan. Bake 1 1/2 hours. Cool.

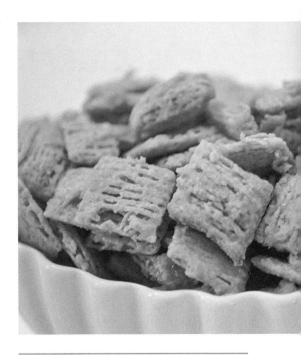

MAKES 6 (1/2-cup) servings

PREP TIME 5 minutes

COOK TIME 1 1/2 hours

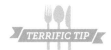
TERRIFIC TIP

You can also toss in nuts or dried fruit.

. . . .

DOC'S NOTE

Keep this on hand for daily snacking. Every calorie counts. Peanut butter adds protein and the cereal adds fiber, vitamins, and minerals.

NUTRITIONAL INFORMATION Calories 148, Calories from Fat 25%, Fat 4 g, Saturated Fat 1 g, Cholesterol 0 mg, Sodium 77 mg, Carbohydrates 26 g, Dietary Fiber 3 g, Total Sugars 7 g, Protein 4 g

DIABETIC EXCHANGES 1 1/2 starch, 1/2 other carbohydrate, 1/2 fat

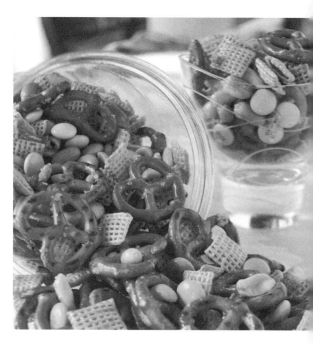

SNACK MIX

An irresistible sweet-and-salty combination creates this favorite munch mix.

3 tablespoons sesame oil
3 tablespoons honey
1 tablespoon low-sodium soy sauce
1 teaspoon garlic powder
4 cups honey-nut toasted rice and corn cereal squares
6 cups mini-pretzels
1 cup dry roasted peanuts
1 cup candy-coated chocolate pieces

1 Preheat oven 250°F. Line baking pan with foil.

2 In small bowl, whisk together sesame oil, honey, soy sauce, and garlic powder.

3 On prepared pan, combine cereal squares, pretzels, and peanuts. Add oil mixture and toss with cereal mixture. Bake 25 minutes, stirring once.

4 Turn off oven and leave in oven 1 hour to continue crisping. Cool completely and toss with chocolate candies. Store in an airtight container.

MAKES 20 (1/2-cup) servings
PREP TIME 10 minutes
COOK TIME 25 minutes + 1 hour to crisp

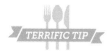

Pre-portion out into plastic zip-top bags to grab for an easy snack on-the-go. Use seasonal chocolate candies for the different holidays.

. . . .

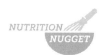

Fortified cereals provide a host of nutrients including calcium, iron, fiber, folic acid, and vitamins C, B, and A.

NUTRITIONAL INFORMATION Calories 205, Calories from Fat 36%, Fat 8 g, Saturated Fat 2 g, Cholesterol 1 mg, Sodium 357 mg, Carbohydrates 29 g, Dietary Fiber 1 g, Total Sugars 12 g, Protein 4 g

DIABETIC EXCHANGES 2 starch, 1 fat

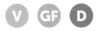

NO-BAKE ENERGY BITES

These bites with oatmeal, coconut, peanut butter and chocolate chips pack a subtlety sweet, yet filling taste of goodness.

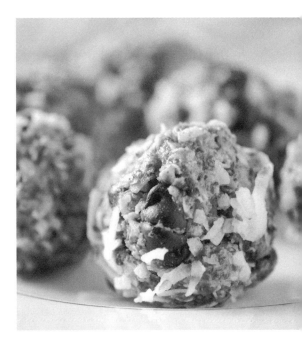

1 cup old-fashioned oatmeal
1/3 cup toasted coconut
1/2 cup peanut butter
1/2 cup ground flaxseed
1/2 cup dark chocolate chips (optional)
1/3 cup honey
1 teaspoon vanilla extract

1. In medium bowl, stir together all ingredients until thoroughly mixed. Refrigerate 30 minutes or until well chilled.

2. Once chilled, roll into heaping teaspoon-size balls. Store in airtight container and keep refrigerated up to 1 week.

MAKES 25 balls

PREP TIME 30 minutes (in refrigerator)

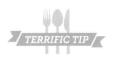

These stay fresh in an airtight container in the refrigerator for up to a week, so make ahead and snack on when feeling low in energy.

· · · · · · · · · · · · · · · ·

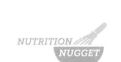

If adding chocolate chips, try dark chocolate chips for added antioxidants.

NUTRITIONAL INFORMATION Calories 74, Calories from Fat 46%, Fat 4 g, Saturated Fat 1 g, Cholesterol 0 mg, Sodium 28 mg, Carbohydrates 8 g, Dietary Fiber 1 g, Total Sugars 5 g, Protein 2 g

DIABETIC EXCHANGES 1/2 other carbohydrate, 1 fat

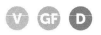

GRANOLA BARS

Easy-to-make yummy bars with toasted oatmeal and honey mixture combined with your favorite ingredients.

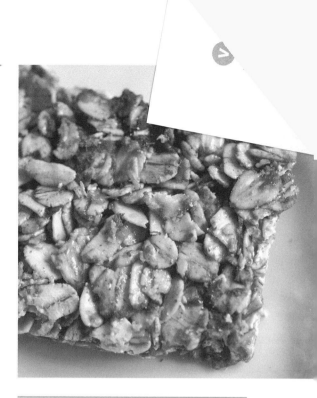

3 cups old-fashioned oatmeal
2 tablespoons oil
2 tablespoons light brown sugar
2 tablespoons maple syrup
1/4 cup honey
1 teaspoon vanilla extract
1 teaspoon cinnamon
1 cup assorted ingredients (dark chocolate chips, nuts, cranberries, raisins, sunflower seeds)

1 Preheat oven 350°F. Line baking pan with foil.

2 Spread oatmeal evenly on pan. Bake about 15 minutes, stirring once; until slightly golden (smell toasty oats).

3 In microwave-safe dish, mix together oil, brown sugar, maple syrup, honey, vanilla, and cinnamon. Microwave 2 minutes or until bubbly and brown sugar dissolved. Line 9×9×2-inch pan with large piece of foil that comes up the sides and covers the top.

4 In large bowl, combine toasted oatmeal with honey mixture, stirring to coat evenly. Stir in 1 cup assorted ingredients. Transfer mixture into prepared pan. Fold foil over top of granola in pan and press to fill corners and flatten granola to fit pan evenly. Cool at least an hour, or can refrigerate or freeze to set faster.

5 Lift out of pan holding foil and slice down middle and cut each half into 8 bars.

MAKES 16 bars
PREP TIME 15 minutes
COOK TIME 15 minutes + time to cool

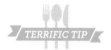

Keep these pantry friendly ingredients on hand for a quick satisfying snack.

• • • • • • • • • • • • • • • •

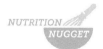

A gluten-free diet has been shown to reduce adiposity gain, inflammation and insulin resistance.

NUTRITIONAL INFORMATION Calories 150, Calories from Fat 33%, Fat 6 g, Saturated Fat 1 g, Cholesterol 0 mg, Sodium 1 mg, Carbohydrates 23 g, Dietary Fiber 2 g, Total Sugars 12 g, Protein 3 g
DIABETIC EXCHANGES 1 starch, 1/2 other carbohydrate, 1 fat

GUACAMAME

Avocado and edamame magically create this incredible creamy, tasty and nutritious dip. Serve with fresh veggies or pita chips.

1 large avocado, (about 2/3 cup mashed)
1 1/2 cups shelled edamame, thawed
2 tablespoons lime juice
1/2 teaspoon minced garlic
1/2 cup salsa
3 tablespoons nonfat plain Greek yogurt
Salt and pepper to taste

1 In food processor, combine all ingredients, mixing until smooth.

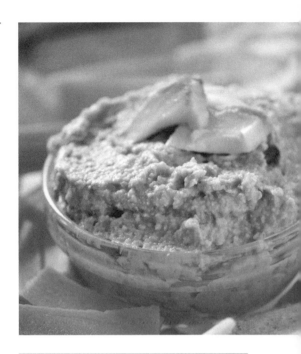

MAKES 10 (1/4-cup) servings
PREP TIME 10 minutes

TERRIFIC TIP

Use to stuff vegetables or as a sandwich spread.

DOC'S NOTE

Soybeans are high in omega 3 fatty acids, which are necessary to ingest through food for their anti-inflammatory benefits.

NUTRITIONAL INFORMATION Calories 62, Calories from Fat 47%, Fat 3 g, Saturated Fat 0 g, Cholesterol 0 mg, Sodium 50 mg, Carbohydrates 5 g, Dietary Fiber 2 g, Total Sugars 2 g, Protein 4 g
DIABETIC EXCHANGES 1 vegetable, 1/2 fat

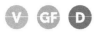

MEDITERRANEAN LAYERED DIP

My most requested Greek captivating layered dip with hummus and fresh veggies. Keep in the refrigerator to munch on all week. Serve with pita chips or raw vegetables.

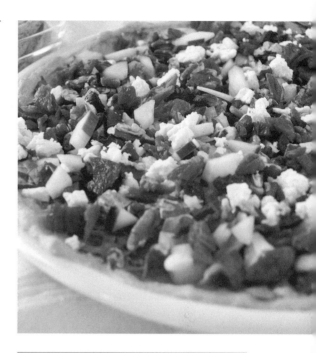

1 (7-ounce) container hummus
1 cup coarsely chopped fresh baby spinach
1/2 cup chopped tomatoes
1/2 cup chopped cucumber
1/4 cup chopped red onion
1/4 cup crumbled reduced-fat feta cheese
2 tablespoons sliced Kalamata or black olives

1 Spread hummus on 9-inch serving plate.

2 Sprinkle evenly with remaining ingredients, refrigerate until serving time.

MAKES 8 (1/3-cup) servings
PREP TIME 15 minutes

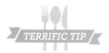

Look for different containers of flavored hummus (I love roasted red pepper) to give this recipe extra punch. Raid a salad or olive bar for quality olives in the amount you need.

· · · · · · · · · · · · · · · ·

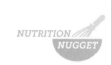

Hummus is a nutrient dense source of protein and fiber.

NUTRITIONAL INFORMATION Calories 61, Calories from Fat 31%, Fat 3 g, Saturated Fat 1 g, Cholesterol 2 mg, Sodium 189 mg, Carbohydrates 5 g, Dietary Fiber 2 g, Total Sugars 1 g, Protein 3 g
DIABETIC EXCHANGES 1/2 starch, 1/2 fat

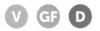

STRAWBERRY FRUIT DIP

Wonderful dip to keep in the refrigerator to serve with your favorite fruits.

1 quart strawberries, stemmed and finely chopped
2 tablespoons light brown sugar
1/4 cup orange juice
1 cup nonfat vanilla Greek yogurt
1/2 teaspoon grated orange rind, optional

1 In bowl, mix together all ingredients. Refrigerate.

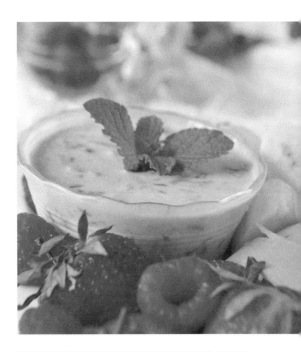

MAKES 40 (1-tablespoon) servings

PREP TIME 10 minutes

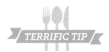
TERRIFIC TIP

If trying to gain weight use full fat yogurt, add dry milk powder or add tofu. Try different flavored yogurts.

DOC'S NOTE

Get your extra potassium and vitamin C from strawberries. If white blood cell count is low, don't use raw fruit to make dip.

NUTRITIONAL INFORMATION Calories 13, Calories from Fat 0%, Fat 0 g, Saturated Fat 0 g, Cholesterol 0 mg, Sodium 2 mg, Carbohydrates 3 g, Dietary Fiber 0 g, Total Sugars 2 g, Protein 1 g

DIABETIC EXCHANGES Free

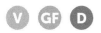

KALE CHIPS

Crisp and crunchy; melts in your mouth.
No-fuss, simple, easy-to-eat recipe.

1 bunch of curly kale, washed, dried,
  torn into 2-inch pieces
Salt to taste

1 Preheat oven 400°F. Line baking pan with foil
   and coat with nonstick cooking spray.

2 Spread kale on prepared pan in single layer.
   Coat kale lightly with nonstick cooking spray.
   Season to taste.

3 Bake 8–10 minutes or until kale is crispy and
   edges brown.

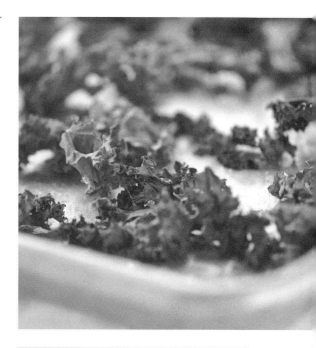

MAKES **8 servings**
PREP TIME **5 minutes**
COOK TIME **10 minutes**

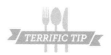
TERRIFIC TIP

Look for chopped kale in
bags at the grocery.

· · · · · · · · · · · · · · · · ·

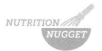
NUTRITION NUGGET

Did you know kale is a good
source of calcium; the most
abundant mineral in the body.

NUTRITIONAL INFORMATION Calories 19, Calories from Fat 0%, Fat 0 g, Saturated Fat 0 g, Cholesterol 0 mg,
Sodium 17 mg, Carbohydrates 4 g, Dietary Fiber 1 g, Total Sugars 0 g, Protein 1 g

DIABETIC EXCHANGES Free

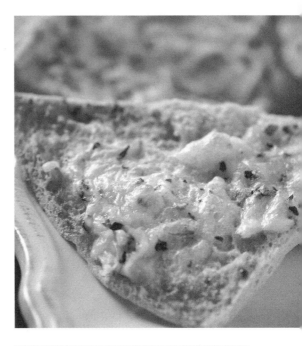

V **D**

PARMESAN PITAS

These fantastic, crispy seasoned pitas (like chips) may be eaten warm or room temperature. Sometimes crunchy pick-ups are good to have on hand.

1/2 cup light mayonnaise
1/4 cup nonfat plain yogurt
3/4 cup grated Parmesan cheese
1 teaspoon dried basil leaves
1 teaspoon dried oregano leaves
1 teaspoon lemon juice
5 whole pita breads (whole-wheat)

1 Preheat oven 350°F. Coat baking pan with nonstick cooking spray.

2 In small bowl, mix together all ingredients except pita bread.

3 Split pita bread in half and cut each whole into six triangles (each pita makes 12 triangles). Spread each triangle with about 1/2 teaspoon mixture. Bake 8–10 minutes or until crispy.

MAKES 15 (4-triangle) servings
PREP TIME 15 minutes
COOK TIME 10 minutes

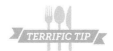
TERRIFIC TIP

Use kitchen scissors to easily cut pitas. Italian seasoning blend may be substituted for basil and oregano or change the seasoning to your desired herbs.

· · · · · · · · · · · · · · · · ·

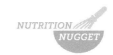
NUTRITION NUGGET

By choosing whole-wheat pita bread you are increasing your fiber intake by 4 grams per pita.

NUTRITIONAL INFORMATION Calories 92, Calories from Fat 33%, Fat 4 g, Saturated Fat 1 g, Cholesterol 0 mg, Sodium 6 mg, Carbohydrates 12 g, Dietary Fiber 1 g, Total Sugars 1 g, Protein 4 g
DIABETIC EXCHANGES 1 starch, 1/2 fat

MEATY MEDITERRANEAN PITA NACHOS

Crispy pita chips layered with cool cucumber sauce and fresh Mediterranean ingredients.

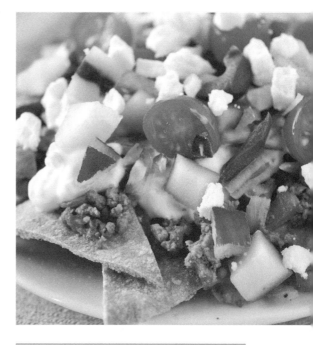

6 whole-wheat pitas, split and each half cut into 8 triangles
1/2 pound ground sirloin
1/2 cup chopped onion
1/2 teaspoon minced garlic
1/2 teaspoon cumin
1/2 cup chopped red onion

1/2 cup grape tomatoes, sliced in half
1/2 cup chopped cucumber
1/3 cup reduced-fat crumbled feta
3 tablespoons sliced Kalamata olives

1 Preheat oven 400°F. Coat baking pan with nonstick cooking spray. Lay pita triangles on baking sheet and bake about 10 minutes or until crispy.

3 In nonstick skillet, cook meat, onion, and garlic until meat is done. Add cumin; set aside.

4 Arrange crispy pitas on plate. Spread meat over pitas and top with Tzatziki Sauce and sprinkle with red onion, tomatoes, cucumber, feta and olives.

TZATZIKI SAUCE

1 cup nonfat plain Greek yogurt
1/2 cup peeled and seeded finely diced cucumber

1 teaspoon minced garlic
1 teaspoon white wine vinegar
1 tablespoon lemon juice
Salt and pepper to taste

1 In small bowl, combine all ingredients.

MAKES 8 servings
PREP TIME 15 minutes
COOK TIME 15 minutes

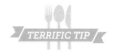
TERRIFIC TIP

Take a short cut and buy pita chips instead of making them. Also, may be served as a meal. Tzatziki Sauce also makes a great dip.

. . . .

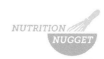
NUTRITION NUGGET

Greek yogurt is an excellent low-fat, low-sugar, high-protein substitute for plain yogurt or sour cream.

NUTRITIONAL INFORMATION Calories 209, Calories from Fat 18%, Fat 4 g, Saturated Fat 1 g, Cholesterol 17 mg, Sodium 412 mg, Carbohydrates 30 g, Dietary Fiber 4 g, Total Sugars 3 g, Protein 15 g

DIABETIC EXCHANGES 2 starch, 1 1/2 lean meat

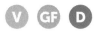

SPINACH SALAD WITH APPLES AND ORANGES
WITH CITRUS VINAIGRETTE

A refreshing crisp fruity spinach salad with the perfect crunch of apples, celery and tangy oranges, complemented by the citrus vinaigrette can make a nice light meal or snack.

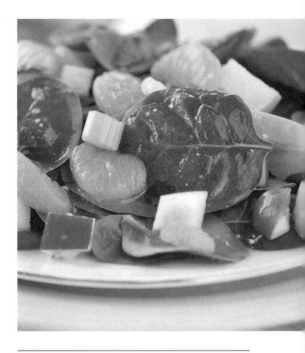

1 (6-ounce) package fresh baby spinach (6 cups baby spinach)
1 cup chopped red apples
1 cup chopped green apples
1 cup chopped celery
1 (11-ounce) can mandarin oranges, drained and reserving 3 tablespoons mandarin juice
Citrus Vinaigrette (recipe follows)

MAKES 6 servings

PREP TIME 15 minutes

1 In large bowl, combine spinach, red and green apples, celery and oranges.

2 Toss salad with Citrus Vinaigrette and serve.

CITRUS VINAIGRETTE

1/2 teaspoon Dijon mustard
Salt and pepper to taste
2 tablespoons lemon juice
3 tablespoons reserved mandarin juice
2 tablespoons honey
2 tablespoons olive oil

1 In a small bowl, whisk together all ingredients.

TERRIFIC TIP

Top with grilled chicken or shrimp for an entrée salad and protein.

· · · · · · · · · · · · · · · · ·

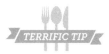
NUTRITION
NUGGET

6 cups uncooked spinach equals 1 cup cooked— that's 6 cups of nutrients packed into 1!

NUTRITIONAL INFORMATION Calories 113, Calories from Fat 40%, Fat 5 g, Saturated Fat 1 g, Cholesterol 0 mg, Sodium 42 mg, Carbohydrates 19 g, Dietary Fiber 3 g, Total Sugars 15 g, Protein 2 g

DIABETIC EXCHANGES 1 carbohydrate, 1 fat

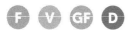

SPINACH AND CHEESE TORTILLA PIZZA

Who says you can't have a quick pizza? Whip up this easy, delightful tortilla pizza.

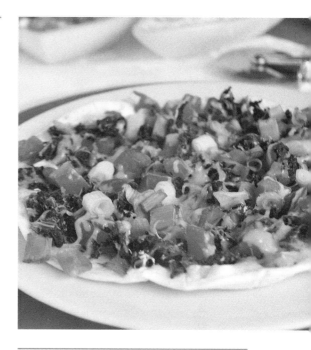

2 (10-inch) flour tortillas (corn tortillas for gluten-free)
2 tablespoons nonfat plain Greek yogurt
1 (10-ounce) package frozen chopped spinach, thawed and squeezed dry
1 large tomato, chopped
1/2 cup shredded reduced-fat Mexican blend cheese
1/4 cup chopped green onions

1 Preheat oven 450°F. Coat baking pan with nonstick cooking spray.

2 Place tortillas on baking sheet. Bake 2 minutes, or until golden brown. Remove from oven and reduce temperature 350°F.

3 Spread yogurt evenly over tortillas. Top with spinach and tomato and sprinkle with cheese.

4 Return to oven 5 minutes more or until cheese is melted. Sprinkle with green onions. Cut each tortilla into 6 slices.

MAKES 12 slices
PREP TIME 10 minutes
COOK TIME 7 minutes

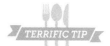

Keep ingredients in refrigerator for quick last minute snack. Top with your favorite ingredients.

· · · · · · · · · · · · · · · · ·

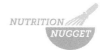

Use corn tortillas for a gluten-free option.

NUTRITIONAL INFORMATION Calories 64, Calories from Fat 25%, Fat 2 g, Saturated Fat 1 g, Cholesterol 3 mg, Sodium 108 mg, Carbohydrates 9 g, Dietary Fiber 1 g, Total Sugars 1 g, Protein 3 g
DIABETIC EXCHANGES 1/2 starch

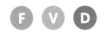

CHEESE QUESADILLAS

Easy to prepare and add other ingredients you feel like eating.

2 (6–8-inch) flour or corn tortillas
1/2 cup shredded reduced-fat Cheddar or Mexican blend cheese
Salsa or taco sauce, if desired

1 In pan coated with nonstick cooking spray, place one tortilla. Sprinkle with cheese and top with other tortilla. Cook about 1–1 1/2 minutes on each side, over low heat, turning with a spatula.

2 Coat pan again with nonstick cooking spray, and use spatula to turn, cooking until cheese melted and tortillas are light brown. Watch carefully.

3 Cut into six wedges, and serve with salsa or taco sauce, if desired.

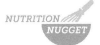

NUTRITION NUGGET

Snacking is strongly encouraged when trying to maintain weight, as light meals and snacks are often better tolerated than large meals. You can add leftover rotisserie chicken for a lean meat, high protein option.

NUTRITIONAL INFORMATION Calories 110, Calories from Fat 28%, Fat 3 g, Saturated Fat 2 g, Cholesterol 10 mg, Sodium 294 mg, Carbohydrates 12 g, Dietary Fiber 1 g, Total Sugars 0 g, Protein 7 g

DIABETIC EXCHANGES 1 starch, 1/2 lean meat

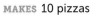

MINI CHEESE PIZZAS

Sometimes a simple pizza hits the spot! Here's an easy-to-make super quick snack or light lunch.

1 (10-biscuit) can flaky refrigerated biscuits
1/3 cup tomato sauce
1/2 teaspoon dried oregano leaves
1/2 cup shredded part-skim mozzarella cheese

1 Preheat oven 450°F. Coat baking pan with nonstick cooking spray.

2 Pat each biscuit into 4-inch circle on prepared pan.

3 In small bowl, mix tomato sauce and oregano. Spoon sauce on each biscuit round.

4 Sprinkle cheese over tomato sauce. Bake 8-10 minutes or until cheese is melted.

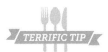

TERRIFIC TIP

Keep in the fridge to pop out when you want a snack or light meal. Look for whole-wheat biscuits. Add seasonings or veggies to preference, such as bell peppers, black olives, and mushrooms for extra vitamins and nutrients.

NUTRITIONAL INFORMATION Calories 70, Calories from Fat 8%, Fat 2 g, Saturated Fat 1 g, Cholesterol 4 mg, Sodium 257 mg, Carbohydrates 10 g, Dietary Fiber 0 g, Total Sugars 1 g, Protein 3 g

DIABETIC EXCHANGES 1/2 starch, 1/2 fat

F **GF** **D**

SWEET POTATO SKINS

This all-American favorite gets a deliciously healthy spin with fiber-rich sweet potatoes and healthier ingredients, ideal for an amazing snack or light meal.

6 medium sweet potatoes
4 slices turkey bacon, cooked and crumbled, optional
1/2 cup chopped green onions
2/3 cup reduced-fat shredded Cheddar cheese

1 Wash potatoes well, and dry thoroughly. Microwave on high 8–10 minutes depending on size (or oven bake at 425°F for 50–60 minutes). When potatoes are cool to handle, cut in half lengthwise. Scoop out the pulp, leaving a 1/4-inch shell. (Save pulp for use in another recipe, see Terrific Tip.) Cut potato skins in half width-wise.

2 Place potato skins on baking pan lined with foil. Coat skins with nonstick cooking spray.

3 Bake 475°F for 5–7 minutes; turn and coat skins on other side with nonstick cooking spray. Bake until crisp, 3–5 minutes more.

4 In small bowl, mix together bacon, if desired, green onions, and cheese. Sprinkle mixture inside skins. Bake 2 minutes longer or until cheese is melted.

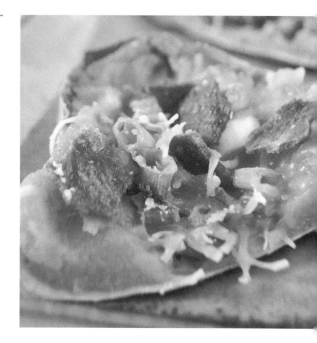

MAKES 12 potato skins
PREP TIME 15 minutes
COOK TIME 25 minutes

TERRIFIC TIP

With the extra potato pulp, make mashed sweet potatoes by mixing in skim milk, sour cream, salt and pepper and maybe a dash of cinnamon.

• • • • • • • • • • • • • • • • • •

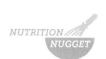

NUTRITION
NUGGET

Sweet potato skin is full of nutrition, including fiber and beta-carotene; which converts to vitamin A—an antioxidant powerhouse.

NUTRITIONAL INFORMATION Calories 65, Calories from Fat 16%, Fat 1 g, Saturated Fat 1 g, Cholesterol 3 mg, Sodium 71 mg, Carbohydrates 11 g, Dietary Fiber 2 g, Total Sugars 2 g, Protein 3 g
DIABETIC EXCHANGES 1 starch

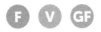

PEANUT BUTTER SNACK PIE

If you have a sweet tooth, but don't want anything too sweet, this yummy crustless pie makes a light peanut butter treat.

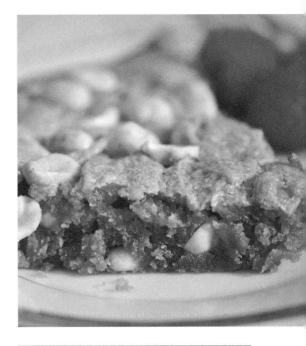

1/2 cup light brown sugar
2 eggs
2 teaspoons vanilla extract
3/4 cup peanut butter
3/4 cup chopped peanuts

1 Preheat oven 350°F.

2 In bowl, whisk together brown sugar, eggs and vanilla. Blend in peanut butter and stir in peanuts.

3 Spread batter evenly into pan. Bake 20–25 minutes or just until pie is set.

MAKES 10 servings
PREP TIME 10 minutes
COOK TIME 25 minutes

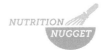
TERRIFIC TIP

Add dark chocolate chips for a chocolate peanut butter snack pie. If you have a sore mouth, leave out the peanuts.

. . . .

NUTRITION
NUGGET

Peanuts actually belong to the legume family, which includes beans and lentils rather than being a true nut. Peanuts are nutritionally and calorically dense, being high in healthy monounsaturated fat, as well as vitamin E.

NUTRITIONAL INFORMATION Calories 237, Calories from Fat 58%, Fat 16 g, Saturated Fat 3 g, Cholesterol 37 mg, Sodium 102 mg, Carbohydrates 17 g, Dietary Fiber 2 g, Total Sugars 13 g, Protein 8 g

DIABETIC EXCHANGES 1 other carbohydrate, 1 lean meat, 2 1/2 fat

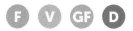

PEACHY PEAR REFRESHER

A refreshing smoothie-style drink with a subtle zing.

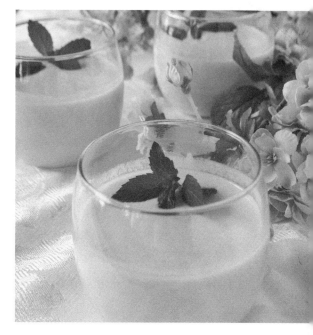

1 pear, peeled and coarsely chopped (1 cup)
1/2 cup nonfat peach yogurt
1/2 cup pear nectar
1 teaspoon lime juice
1/4 teaspoon ground ginger
1/2 cup small ice cubes

1 In food processor or blender, blend all ingredients until smooth.

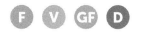

MAKES 4 (2/3 cup) servings

PEACH SMOOTHIE

This velvety, exceptionally easy and delicious peach recipe makes a great smoothie or a soup.

1 (14-ounce) can sliced peaches, drained
1 cup nonfat vanilla Greek yogurt
1 cup orange juice or peach nectar
1 teaspoon lemon juice
2 teaspoons sugar, optional
1 teaspoon almond extract

1 In food processor or blender, blend all ingredients until smooth.

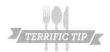

TERRIFIC TIP

Freeze extra smoothie to thaw for a quick snack another day. Frozen or fresh peaches may be subsituted for canned.

DOC'S NOTE

Pears are a great source of fiber, as well as a good source of vitamin C. The yellow-orange color of peaches indicates they are rich in beta-carotene, protecting the body against free radicals.

PEACHY PEAR REFRESHER NUTRITIONAL INFORMATION Calories 151, Calories from Fat 0%, Fat 0 g, Saturated Fat 0 g, Cholesterol 6 mg, Sodium 55 mg, Carbohydrates 35 g, Dietary Fiber 4 g, Total Sugars 27 g, Protein 5 g

DIABETIC EXCHANGES 2 carbohydrate

PEAR SMOOTHIE NUTRITIONAL INFORMATION Calories 119, Calories from Fat 0%, Fat 0 g, Saturated Fat 0, Cholesterol 0 mg, Sodium 20 mg, Carbohydrates 24 g, Dietary Fiber 1 g, Total Sugars 21 g, Protein 5 g

DIABETIC EXCHANGES 1 fruit, 1/2 fat-free milk

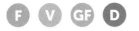

MANGO PINEAPPLE SMOOTHIE

With all frozen ingredients, this delicious smoothie whips up in minutes.

1 cup frozen mango chunks
1 cup frozen pineapple chunks
1/2 cup skim milk
1/2 cup nonfat vanilla Greek yogurt
1 banana, frozen (time permitted)

1 In food processor or blender, blend all ingredients until smooth.

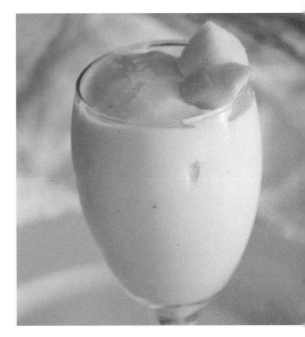

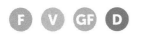

MAKES 2 (1-cup) serving

WATERMELON SLUSH

Cool and refreshing for a sore mouth.

1 cup ice
2 cups watermelon chunks, seeded
2 tablespoons honey

1 In food processor or blender, blend all ingredients until smooth.

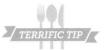

Use ice as tolerated, since cool and room temperature food and drinks are sometimes better tolerated than very cold and very hot foods.

Watermelon is an excellent source of vitamin C, vitamin A, and the antioxidant, lycopene.

MANGO PINEAPPLE SMOOTHIE NUTRITIONAL INFORMATION Calories 214, Calories from Fat 3%, Fat 1 g, Saturated Fat 0 g, Cholesterol 1 mg, Sodium 44 mg, Carbohydrates 47 g, Dietary Fiber 4 g, Total Sugars 36 g, Protein 8 g

DIABETIC EXCHANGES 2 fruit, 1 fat-free milk

WATERMELON SLUSH NUTRITIONAL INFORMATION Calories 109, Calories from Fat 6%, Fat 0 g, Saturated Fat 0 g, Cholesterol 0 mg, Sodium 2 mg, Carbohydrates 29 g, Dietary Fiber 1 g, Total Sugars 27 g, Protein 1 g

DIABETIC EXCHANGES 1 fruit, 1 other carbohydrate

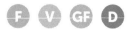

BERRY SMOOTHIE

Refreshing, soothing, and wonderful.

- 1 cup strawberries, fresh or frozen
- 1/2 cup blueberries
- 1 tablespoon sugar
- 1/4 cup skim milk
- 1/4 cup nonfat vanilla Greek yogurt

1 In food processor or blender, blend all ingredients until smooth.

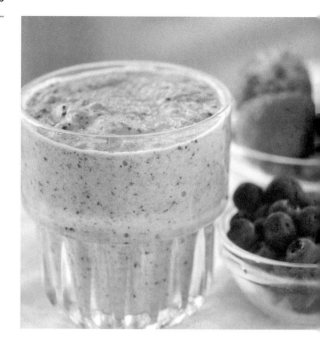

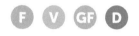

MAKES 2 servings

TROPICAL SMOOTHIE

Smoothies are a great food substitute when you don't have an appetite.

- 1 ripe banana, sliced
- 1/2 cup chopped peaches (fresh or frozen)
- 1 cup mango, papaya, peach nectar or juice
- 1/2 cup milk (any type) or nutritional energy drink supplement
- 4 ice cubes

1 In food processor or blender, blend all ingredients until smooth.

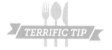
TERRIFIC TIP

In any smoothie recipe, use whichever liquid you prefer: soy milk, rice milk, almond milk, oat milk, regular nonfat milk or liquid nutritional supplements.

. . . .

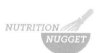
NUTRITION NUGGET

Greek yogurt is a high protein, low sugar version of yogurt. Bananas offer loads of important nutrients to help build collagen and beat inflammation such as vitamin C, B-6 and folate.

BERRY SMOOTHIE NUTRITIONAL INFORMATION Calories 99, Calories from Fat 0%, Fat 0 g, Saturated Fat 0 g, Cholesterol 0 mg, Sodium 27 mg, Carbohydrates 21 g, Dietary Fiber 3 g, Total Sugars 17 g, Protein 4 g

DIABETIC EXCHANGES 1 1/2 carbohydrate, 1/2 fat-free milk

TROPICAL SMOOTHIE NUTRITIONAL INFORMATION Calories 165, Calories from Fat 0%, Fat 0 g, Saturated Fat 0 g, Cholesterol 1 mg, Sodium 29 mg, Carbohydrates 40 g, Dietary Fiber 3 g, Total Sugars 32 g, Protein 3 g

DIABETIC EXCHANGES 2 1/2 fruit

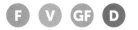

PINEAPPLE GREEN SMOOTHIE

Frozen pineapple keeps this smoothie cold, banana and yogurt make it creamy, and spinach is a green boost of nutrition.

- 1 cup pineapple juice
- 1 1/2 cups fresh baby spinach
- 1 banana
- 1 cup cubed frozen pineapple
- 1/2 cup nonfat vanilla or flavored Greek yogurt

1 In food processor or blender, blend all ingredients until smooth.

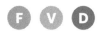

MAKES 2 (1-cup) serving

GREEN SMOOTHIE

Fresh and invigorating, great and satisfying, morning, noon or night.

- 1 cup packed baby spinach
- 1/3 cup coconut water
- 1/3 cup vanilla Greek yogurt
- 1/3 cup skim milk
- Half banana
- 2/3 cup ice

1 In food processor or blender, blend all ingredients until smooth.

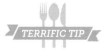
TERRIFIC TIP

Add more liquid to reach desired consistency, or add more ice to thicken.

. . . .

DOC'S NOTE

You know spinach is loaded with healthy nutrients by the rich color green; boasting powerful antioxidant protection—add it to any dish you can—even smoothies! Pineapples have high amounts of manganese, which is important for antioxidant defenses.

PINEAPPLE GREEN SMOOTHIE NUTRITIONAL INFORMATION Calories 219, Calories from Fat 0%, Fat 0 g, Saturated Fat 0 g, Cholesterol 0 mg, Sodium 40 mg, Carbohydrates 49 g, Dietary Fiber 3 g, Total Sugars 35 g, Protein 6 g

DIABETIC EXCHANGES 3 fruit, 1/2 fat-free milk

GREEN SMOOTHIE NUTRITIONAL INFORMATION Calories 79, Calories from fat 3%, Fat 1 g, Saturated Fat 0 g, Cholesterol 1 mg, Sodium 90 mg, Carbohydrates 14 g, Dietary Fiber 2 g, Total Sugars 10 g, Protein 6 g

DIABETIC EXCHANGES 1/2 fruit, 1/2 fat-free milk

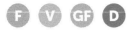

GOOD MORNING SMOOTHIE

A great morning pick-me-up.

1 medium banana
1 cup orange juice
6 ounces low-fat vanilla yogurt
1 cup frozen strawberries

1. In food processor or blender, blend all ingredients until smooth.

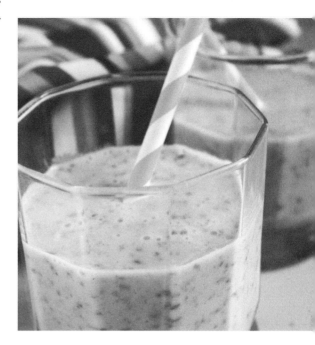

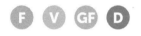

MAKES 2 (1-cup) serving

AWESOME MILKSHAKE

An old-fashioned refreshing milkshake.

1/2 cup skim milk
2 cups frozen nonfat vanilla yogurt or nonfat ice cream
1 teaspoon vanilla extract
3 tablespoons chocolate syrup, optional

1. In food processor or blender, blend all ingredients until smooth. For a chocolate milk shake, add chocolate syrup to the mixture.

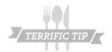

Try using different flavors of yogurt and ice cream to change the taste.

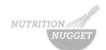

For a more filling smoothie add nut butters like almond or peanut butter as an easy way to add healthy fats and protein. For extra calories, don't use low-fat products and substitute a vanilla nutritional energy drink supplement.

GOOD MORNING SMOOTHIE NUTRITIONAL INFORMATION Calories 110, Calories from Fat 7%, Total Fat 1g, Saturated Fat 0g, Cholesterol 2mg, Sodium 29mg, Total Carbohydrate 24g, Dietary Fiber 2g, Total Sugars 17g, Protein 3g

DIABETIC EXCHANGES 1 fruit, 1/2 fat-free milk

AWESOME MILK SHAKE NUTRITIONAL INFORMATION Calories 218, Calories from Fat 0%, Fat 0 g, Saturated Fat 0 g, Cholesterol 4 mg, Sodium 160 mg, Carbohydrates 41 g, Dietary Fiber 0 g, Total Sugars 41 g, Protein 12 g

DIABETIC EXCHANGES 1/2 skim milk, 2 1/2 other carbohydrate

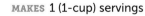

F V

MAKES 1 (1-cup) servings

STRAWBERRY WEIGHT GAIN SHAKE

Freeze the shake in freezer trays for 1 1/2 hours or serve in a glass and stir until desired consistency.

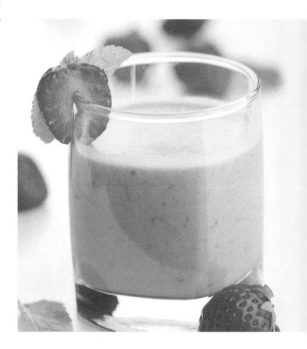

 1 (8-ounce) can vanilla nutritional energy drink supplement, chilled
 1 cup frozen strawberries (unsweetened)
 2 teaspoons sugar

1 In food processor or blender, blend all ingredients until smooth.

F V D

MAKES 1 (1-cup) serving

BASIC WEIGHT GAIN SHAKE

A shake is easy to eat and easy to fix.

 1/2 cup chocolate nutritional energy drink supplement, chilled
 1/2 cup reduced-fat vanilla ice cream

1 In food processor or blender, blend all ingredients until smooth.

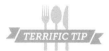

TERRIFIC TIP

Keep frozen mango, pineapple and bananas in the freezer to make when needed. Using a straw to drink liquids and smoothies may help with mouth pain.

· · · · · · · · · · · · · · · · ·

DOC'S NOTE

Great supplement for extra calories; includes vitamins and nutrients.

STRAWBERRY WEIGHT GAIN SHAKE NUTRITIONAL INFORMATION Calories 320, Calories from Fat 12%, Fat 4 g, Saturated Fat 0 g, Cholesterol 0 mg, Sodium 131 mg, Carbohydrates 62 g, Dietary Fiber 3 g, Total Sugars 40 g, Protein 11 g

DIABETIC EXCHANGES 2 1/2 starch, 1 fruit, 1/2 other carbohydrate, 1/2 fat

WEIGHT GAIN SHAKE NUTRITIONAL INFORMATION Calories 228, Calories from Fat 16%, Fat 4 g, Saturated Fat 1 g, Cholesterol 5 mg, Sodium 109 mg, Carbohydrates 39 g, Dietary Fiber 1 g, Total Sugars 25 g, Protein 8 g

DIABETIC EXCHANGES 1/2 very lean meat, 1 1/2 starch, 1 other carb, 1/2 fat

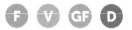

KIWI AND STRAWBERRY SMOOTHIE

A rainbow of green kiwi and strawberry smoothies make a delightfully delicious smoothie. Each smoothie may be served individually.

KIWI SMOOTHIE

3 kiwis
1 banana
1/3 cup nonfat vanilla Greek yogurt
1 cup baby spinach
1 cup skim milk

1 In food processor or blender, blend all ingredients until smooth.

2 Pour 3/4 cup **Kiwi Smoothie** in glass. Top with 1/2 cup **Strawberry Smoothie**. Serve immediately.

STRAWBERRY SMOOTHIE

1 1/2 cups frozen strawberries (unsweetened)
1 banana
1 cup skim milk

1 In food processor or blender, blend all ingredients until smooth.

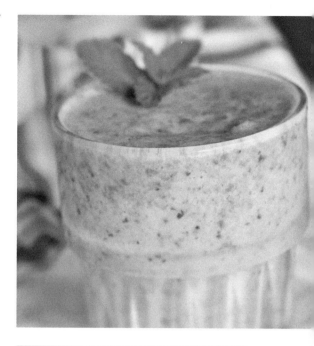

MAKES 4 servings (3/4 cup kiwi layer and 1/2 cup strawberry layer)

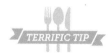

Turn a smoothie into a heartier snack or light dessert, top with granola and diced fresh fruit.

. . . .

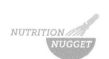

Kiwi and strawberries are packed with vitamin C and are a great fiber source.

NUTRITIONAL INFORMATION Calories 164, Calories from Fat 3%, Fat 1 g, Saturated Fat 0 g, Cholesterol 2 mg, Sodium 66 mg, Carbohydrates 35 g, Dietary Fiber 4 g, Total Sugars 23 g, Protein 7 g

DIABETIC EXCHANGES 2 fruit, 1/2 fat-free milk

CAREGIVER

Easy-to-prepare recipes that freeze well, can be made ahead of time, and served later with minimal preparation.

. . . .

There is nothing more comforting when you are sick than an act of kindness from a friend. Sometimes patients do not want to discuss their appetite or their situation. Being there to listen and offer a warm smile is often the greatest gift. A thoughtful snack, casserole, or other healthy dish can bring joy and happiness to a loved one. Always bring in **disposable, freezable containers** for the patient to eat on their own timeframe. This can also be helpful for family members or caregivers.

The smell of cooking can upset your stomach at times (look at the Nausea section for cold, odorless recipes, page 40). Patients often have their food prepared in an outside kitchen to avoid the aroma. Having a surprise meal will sometimes entice you to eat. We will try to offer recipes for foods that can be heated, defrosted, or served with minimal preparation. A real treat is to include paper plates, forks and spoons so you do not have to worry about washing dishes and your meal really is ready to eat. Try to keep it simple and inviting. Eating with a friend or family can also be very helpful. It is no fun to eat alone.

In this chapter, you will find great recipe suggestions to take to someone or to prepare as a Caregiver.

WHAT CAN PEOPLE DO TO HELP?

- Encourage and support without being overwhelming.
- Accompany you to the grocery store.
- Take your list and go shopping for you.
- Help you to prepare food.
- Help organize ready-to-eat snacks.
- Organize friends or relatives to cook for you and your family.
- Meals should be brought over in disposable containers.
- Run errands for you.
- Eat with you.
- Take you for a ride.
- Read to you.
- Give the caregiver a break.

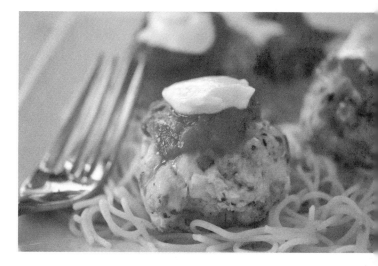

MEXICAN BREAKFAST CASSEROLE

Simple ingredients create this make-ahead scrumptious breakfast dish. Keep in refrigerator to enjoy all week.

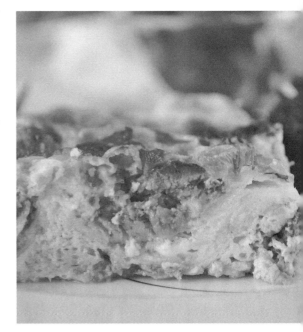

1 (4-ounce) can green chilies

8 ounces ground breakfast turkey sausage

1 onion, chopped

1 red, green, or yellow bell pepper, cored and chopped

1 teaspoon minced garlic

1 tablespoon chili powder

5 eggs

4 egg whites

2 cups fat-free half-and-half

1/2 cup chopped green onions

1 1/2 cups reduced-fat shredded Mexican blend cheese

5 (8-inch) 98% fat-free flour tortillas, cut into fourths (corn tortillas for gluten-free)

1 Coat 13×9×2-inch baking dish with nonstick cooking spray. Spread green chilies along bottom of dish.

2 In large nonstick skillet, cook and crumble sausage until starts to brown. Add onion and bell pepper, cooking until sausage is done and vegetables tender. Add garlic and chili powder. Remove from heat.

3 In large bowl, whisk together eggs, egg whites, and half-and-half. In another bowl, combine green onions and cheese.

4 Spoon one-third of sausage mixture over chilies in baking dish. Top with one-third tortilla quarters and one-third cheese mixture. Repeat layers, ending with cheese. Pour egg mixture evenly over casserole and refrigerate, covered, at least 6 hours or overnight.

5 Preheat oven 350°F. If using glass baking dish, place in cold oven. Bake 50-60 minutes or until bubbly and golden brown. Knife inserted into custard should come out clean.

MAKES 8–10 servings

PREP TIME 25 minutes + time to refrigerate

COOK TIME 1 hour

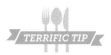
TERRIFIC TIP

Put ingredients together the night before and pop in the oven the next morning for an easy hot breakfast. Adjust the ingredients to your taste buds.

. . . .

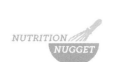
NUTRITION **NUGGET**

Breakfast foods are sometimes better tolerated when not feeling well so enjoy any time of day.

NUTRITIONAL INFORMATION Calories 262, Calories from fat 28%, Fat 7 g, Saturated Fat 3 g, Cholesterol 129 mg, Sodium 578 mg, Carbohydrate 23 g, Dietary Fiber 2 g, Total Sugars 5 g, Protein 18 g

DIABETIC EXCHANGES 1 1/2 starch, 2 1/2 lean meat

(V) (D)

BRUSCHETTA WITH TOMATOES

I think I created the best ever recipe for bruschetta, a fresh, simple and delicious mixture of tomatoes, basil and Kalamatas from the olive bar.

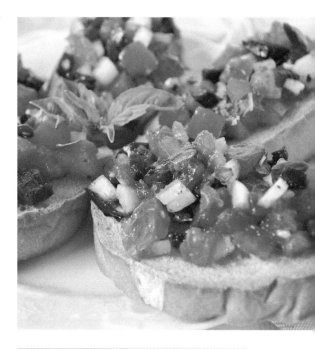

1 loaf French bread
Garlic cloves or minced garlic
1 1/2 cups finely chopped tomatoes (about
  1 1/2 pounds, seeded)
1/4 cup chopped Kalamata olives
1/4 cup chopped onion
2 teaspoons olive oil
1 teaspoon balsamic vinegar
5–6 fresh basil leaves, chopped or 1 teaspoon
  dried basil leaves

1 Preheat oven 450°F. Slice French bread into thin slices and bake about 10 minutes or until crispy. Remove from oven and rub garlic clove across top.

2 In bowl, combine all remaining ingredients. When ready to serve, top toasted bread with tomato mixture.

MAKES 16 servings (bread with about 2 tablespoons topping)
PREP TIME 15 minutes
COOK TIME 10 minutes

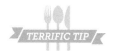

Ahead of time, toast bread and make bruschetta mixture to put together for a quick, delicious snack or appetizer on your time frame. Or, take a short cut and pick up toasted rounds to use.

. . . .

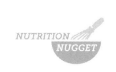

Tomatoes are rich in the mineral potassium.

NUTRITIONAL INFORMATION Calories 97, Calories from fat 16%, Fat 2 g, Saturated Fat 0 g, Cholesterol 0 mg, Sodium 221 mg, Carbohydrate 17 g, Dietary Fiber 1 g, Total Sugars 1 g, Protein 4 g
DIABETIC EXCHANGES 1 starch

TURKEY, BRIE, AND CRANBERRY CHUTNEY QUESADILLAS

Turn leftover holiday turkey into a dinnertime delight with the addition of Brie cheese and cranberry chutney in this easy, fast, and mouth-watering quesadilla.

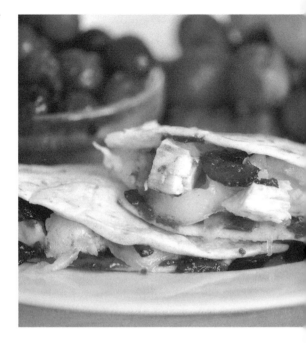

6 (8–10-inch) flour tortillas
1 (9-ounce) jar cranberry chutney
8 ounces Brie cheese, rind removed and sliced
2/3 cup chopped turkey, cooked

1 Preheat oven 425°F. Coat baking pan with nonstick cooking spray.

2 Spread one side of tortilla with cranberry chutney and top with sliced Brie. Add turkey. Fold in half, pressing edges together.

3 Place on prepared pan and bake about 5 minutes or until cheese is melted and tortillas are golden. Let sit a few minutes before cutting into wedges.

MAKES 24 wedges
PREP TIME 10 minutes
COOK TIME 5 minutes

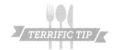

Perfect for leftover holiday food as you can use leftover cranberry sauce and turkey, or make year round with rotisserie chicken.

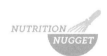

Turkey is an excellent low-calorie high protein food, as 3 ounces provide 25 grams of lean protein.

NUTRITIONAL INFORMATION Calories 85, Calories from Fat 31%, Fat 3 g, Saturated Fat 2 g, Cholesterol 13 mg, Sodium 149 mg, Carbohydrates 10 g, Dietary Fiber 1 g, Total Sugars 4 g, Protein 4 g

DIABETIC EXCHANGES 1/2 starch, 1/2 lean meat

CHICKEN STEW WITH ROASTED BUTTERNUT SQUASH AND QUINOA

A simple, super-satisfying one-pot meal packed with wonderful earthy flavors.

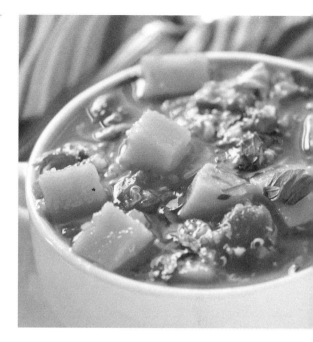

1 1/2 pounds butternut squash, peeled, seeded and chopped into 1/2-inch pieces (about 3 1/2 cups)
1 onion, chopped
2 teaspoons minced garlic
1 (14-ounce) can chopped fire-roasted tomatoes
6 cups low-sodium, fat-free chicken broth
2 teaspoons dried oregano leaves
1/2 cup quinoa
3 cups cooked, chopped skinless chicken breast (rotisserie chicken)
1/4 cup chopped parsley

1. Preheat oven 400°F. Line baking pan with foil and coat with nonstick cooking spray.

2. Spread squash on prepared pan and roast squash 20–25 minutes or until tender and starting to brown.

3. Meanwhile, in large nonstick pot coated with nonstick cooking spray, sauté onion and garlic about 5 minutes; until tender.

4. Add tomatoes, broth, squash, oregano and quinoa. Bring to boil, lower heat and cover, cooking 15 minutes, or until quinoa turns translucent. Add chicken and parsley, heat a few minutes.

MAKES 10 (1-cup) servings
PREP TIME 15 minutes
COOK TIME 45 minutes

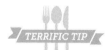

With pre-chopped butternut squash and rotisserie chicken, this recipe is really easy to make.

Quinoa is a grain-like seed that is high in protein, low in fat and also contains iron and fiber—often referred to as a "super grain" due to its high nutritional content.

NUTRITIONAL INFORMATION Calories 147, Calories from Fat 13%, Fat 2g, Saturated Fat 0g, Cholesterol 38mg, Sodium 276mg, Carbohydrates 17g, Dietary Fiber 3g, Total Sugars 4g, Protein 16g
DIABETIC EXCHANGES 1 starch, 2 lean meat

CHICKEN TORTILLA SOUP

This one-pot soup rocks! Make the easy tortilla strips while the soup is cooking.

1 onion, chopped
1 teaspoon minced garlic
1 red bell pepper, cored and chopped
3 corn tortillas, cut into small pieces
5 cups fat-free chicken broth, divided
1 teaspoon ground cumin
1 teaspoon dried oregano leaves
2 cups shredded skinless rotisserie chicken breast
1 cup frozen corn
1 (4-ounce) can green chilies
1 cup red enchilada sauce

1 In large nonstick pot coated with nonstick cooking spray, sauté onion, garlic and bell pepper until tender. Add tortillas and about 1 cup broth, stirring until tortillas are soft and blend into soup

2 Add remaining 4 cups broth and remaining ingredients. Bring to boil, reduce heat, and simmer 15 minutes.

TORTILLA STRIPS

6 (8-inch) flour or corn tortillas (for gluten-free)

1 Preheat oven 350°F. Coat baking pan with nonstick cooking spray.

2 Cut tortillas into thin strips. Spread on prepared pan and bake 15-20 minutes or until lightly browned.

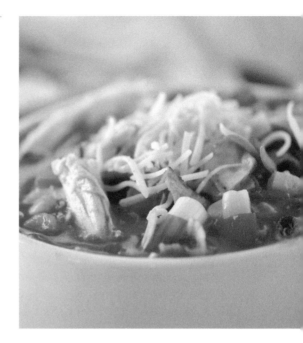

MAKES 8 (1-cup) servings
PREP TIME 20 minutes
COOK TIME 20 minutes

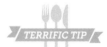

Using corn tortillas flavors and thickens the soup. Serve soup with chopped green onions, cheese, avocado and tortilla strips.

. . . .

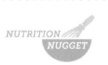

NUTRITION
NUGGET

For a punch of nutrition, toss chopped zucchini and black beans into soup.

SOUP NUTRITIONAL INFORMATION Calories 118, Calories from Fat 16%, Fat 2 g, Saturated Fat 0 g, Cholesterol 32 mg, Sodium 357 mg, Carbohydrates 12 g, Dietary Fiber 2 g, Total Sugars 3 g, Protein 13 g

DIABETIC EXCHANGES 1/2 starch, 1 vegetable, 1 1/2 lean meat

TORTILLA STRIPS NUTRITIONAL INFORMATION Calories 90, Calories from Fat 0%, Fat 0 g, Saturated Fat 0 g, Cholesterol 0 mg, Sodium 255 mg, Carbohydrates 18 g, Dietary Fiber 2 g, Total Sugars 0 g, Protein 3 g

DIABETIC EXCHANGES 1 starch

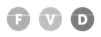

MINESTRONE

A plentiful, fantastic vegetarian one-meal Italian-style vegetable soup. No-salt products reduce the sodium making the recipe diabetic-friendly, but any tomato products may be used.

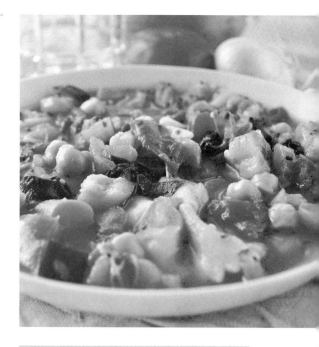

1 onion, chopped
1/2 cup chopped celery
1 teaspoon minced garlic
2 (14 1/2-ounce) cans salt-free diced tomatoes with juice
3 (14-ounce) cans low-sodium vegetable or chicken broth
1 tablespoon dried oregano leaves
1 teaspoon dried basil leaves
1 red potato, peeled and diced
1 cup coarsely chopped carrots
1/2 pound sliced mushrooms
2 cups zucchini, halved lengthwise and thinly sliced
1/3 cup elbow macaroni
1 (16-ounce) cannelloni or white beans, drained and rinsed
1 1/2 cups fresh baby spinach leaves
Salt and pepper to taste

1 In large nonstick pan coated with nonstick cooking spray, sauté onion, celery and garlic until tender. Add diced tomatoes, vegetable broth, oregano, basil, potato, carrots, mushrooms and zucchini. Bring to boil, reduce heat, and cover, cooking 15 minutes.

2 Add pasta and continue cooking another 15 minutes or until pasta is done and vegetables are tender. Stir in beans and spinach, cooking until well heated. Season to taste.

MAKES 10 (1-cup) servings
PREP TIME 20 minutes
COOK TIME 30 minutes

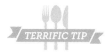
TERRIFIC TIP

Freeze in individual containers to pull out for another meal. Always think about adding extra spinach or vegetables for added nutrition.

DOC'S NOTE

When not feeling well and don't have much of an appetite, eating with a friend or family member can be very helpful and encouraging, as it is no fun to eat alone.

NUTRITIONAL INFORMATION Calories 116, Calories from Fat 0%, Fat 0 g, Saturated Fat 0 g, Cholesterol 0 mg, Sodium 254 mg, Carbohydrates 23 g, Dietary Fiber 5 g, Total Sugars 8 g, Protein 6 g

DIABETIC EXCHANGES 2 vegetable, 1 starch

QUICK SHRIMP AND CORN SOUP

Open up cans of corn and tomatoes, and toss in shrimp for this simple yet superb tomato-based soup.

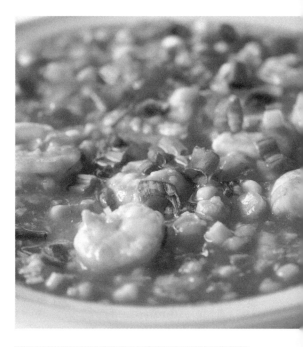

2 (15 1/2-ounce) cans cream-style corn

2 cups frozen corn

2 (14 1/2-ounce) cans diced tomatoes and green chilies

1 (15-ounce) can no-salt tomato sauce

2 pounds medium peeled shrimp

1 bunch green onions, chopped

1 In large nonstick pot, combine cream-style corn, frozen corn, tomatoes and green chilies, and tomato sauce, until heated.

2 Add shrimp, bring to boil. Lower heat, cook until shrimp is done, 5–7 minutes. Sprinkle with green onions, serve.

MAKES 12 (1-cup) servings

PREP TIME 5 minutes

COOK TIME 15 minutes

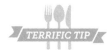
TERRIFIC TIP

Bring in disposable containers and freeze. By using no-salt tomato sauce the recipe is diabetic-friendly, but you can used regular tomato sauce.

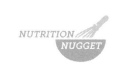
NUTRITION NUGGET

Keep frozen corn in your freezer as a quick fiber-rich addition to many soups, salads and casseroles.

NUTRITIONAL INFORMATION Calories 171, Calories from Fat 6%, Fat 1 g, Saturated Fat 0 g, Cholesterol 122 mg, Sodium 584 mg, Carbohydrates 24 g, Dietary Fiber 4 g, Total Sugars 6 g, Protein 18 g

DIABETIC EXCHANGES 1 1/2 starch, 1 vegetable, 2 lean meat

CRAWFISH PUMPKIN SOUP

Pumpkin and Louisiana crawfish create a simple, snappy smooth soup.

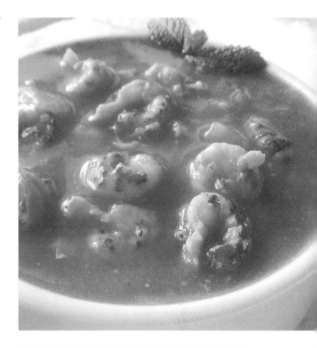

1 onion, chopped
1 (15-ounce) can pumpkin puree
4 cups fat-free chicken broth
1/2 cup skim milk or fat-free half-and-half
1 (16-ounce) bag Louisiana crawfish tails, drained and rinsed
Dash nutmeg
Salt and pepper to taste
1/4 cup chopped green onions

1 In large nonstick pot coated with nonstick cooking spray, sauté onion over medium heat until tender, 5 minutes.

2 Stir in pumpkin and broth, and bring to boil. Reduce heat and simmer 10 minutes. Add milk, crawfish, and nutmeg. Season to taste.

3 Cook over low heat 10 minutes. Serve with green onions.

MAKES **8 (1-cup) servings**
PREP TIME **5 minutes**
COOK TIME **20 minutes**

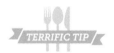
TERRIFIC TIP

The crawfish may be omitted for an easy pumpkin soup.

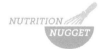
NUTRITION NUGGET

Louisiana crawfish are a good source of protein, vitamins, and minerals; low in calories and fat, especially when rinsed.

NUTRITIONAL INFORMATION Calories 88, Calories from fat 11%, Fat 1 g, Saturated Fat 0 g, Cholesterol 78 mg, Sodium 259 mg, Carbohydrate 7 g, Dietary Fiber 3 g, Total Sugars 4 g, Protein 13 g

DIABETIC EXCHANGES 1/2 starch, 1 1/2 very lean meat

CHICKEN SALAD
WITH CITRUS VINAIGRETTE

Fast and fabulous, this top notch chicken salad features sweet fruit, crunchy cabbage and toasty pecans complemented by a subtle, sweet Citrus Vinaigrette.

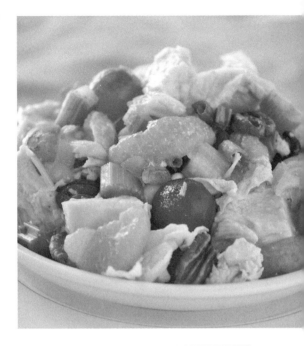

3 cups cooked, diced skinless chicken breasts (rotisserie)
1 cup red grapes, cut in half
1 (11-ounce) can mandarin oranges, drained
1 bunch green onions, chopped
1/3 cup pecan halves, toasted
1/2 cup chopped celery
2 cups shredded Napa cabbage

1 In large bowl, combine chicken, grapes, oranges, green onions, pecans, celery, and cabbage.

2 Toss salad with Citrus Vinaigrette and serve.

CITRUS VINAIGRETTE

2 teaspoons Dijon mustard
Salt and pepper to taste
2 tablespoons lemon juice
2 tablespoons olive oil
1/3 cup orange juice
1 tablespoon honey

1 In a small bowl, whisk together all ingredients.

MAKES **8 (1-cup) servings**
PREP TIME **20 minutes**

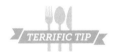
TERRIFIC TIP

Cabbage is an excellent source of vitamin K which is essential in bone health, helping keep calcium in the bones.

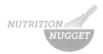
NUTRITION NUGGET

Add seasonal fruits to the salad.

NUTRITIONAL INFORMATION Calories 199, Calories from Fat 39%, Fat 9 g, Saturated Fat 1 g, Cholesterol 47 mg, Sodium 222 mg, Carbohydrates 14 g, Dietary Fiber 2 g, Total Sugars 11 g, Protein 17 g

DIABETIC EXCHANGES 1 fruit, 2 1/2 lean meat

PAELLA SALAD

This festive presentation of colors and textures will quickly convince even the heartiest eaters that a salad can be a satisfying, fulfilling meal.

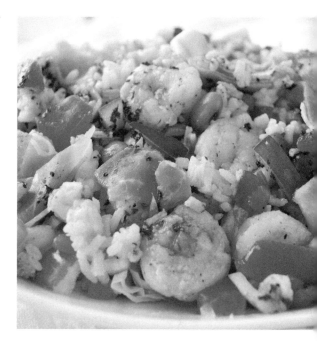

2 (5-ounce) packages yellow rice
1/4 cup balsamic vinegar
1/4 cup lemon juice
1 tablespoon olive oil
1 teaspoon dried basil leaves
1 pound medium cooked and peeled shrimp
1 (14-ounce) can quartered artichoke hearts, drained
3/4 cup chopped green bell pepper
1 cup frozen green peas, thawed
1 cup chopped tomato
1 (2-ounce) jar diced pimiento, drained
1/2 cup chopped red onion
2 ounces chopped prosciutto

1 Prepare rice according to package directions; set aside.

2 In small bowl, mix together vinegar, lemon juice, oil, and basil; set aside.

3 In large bowl, combine cooked rice with shrimp, artichoke hearts, green pepper, peas, tomato, pimiento, red onion, and prosciutto, mixing well.

4 Pour vinaigrette over rice mixture, tossing to coat. Serve or refrigerate until serving.

MAKES **6 servings**
PREP TIME **15 minutes**
COOK TIME **20 minutes**

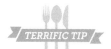

Chicken may be used for shrimp. Great to bring to keep in the refrigerator.

Shrimp are high in selenium, which helps antioxidants fight free radicals, regulate the thyroid gland and may prevent cancer. To make diabetic-friendly, reduce sodium by using white/brown rice for the yellow rice.

NUTRITIONAL INFORMATION Calories 346, Calories from Fat 12%, Fat 4 g, Saturated Fat 1 g, Cholesterol 130 mg, Sodium 817 mg, Carbohydrates 54 g, Dietary Fiber 3 g, Total Sugars 7 g, Protein 25 g

DIABETIC EXCHANGES 2 1/2 lean meat, 3 starch, 1 vegetable

GREEK COUSCOUS SALAD

Don't like to cook? This quick-toss together salad with couscous and Mediterranean ingredients makes a light salad to bring to someone to keep in the refrigerator.

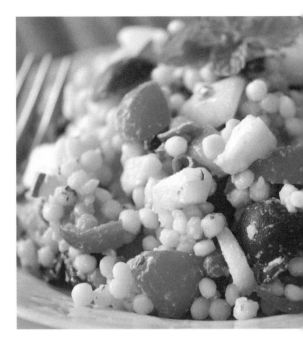

2 cups water
1 1/2 cups Israeli (pearl) couscous or couscous
1 cup chopped tomatoes
1/2 cup chopped cucumbers
1 bunch green onions, chopped
1 cup packed baby spinach
1/3 cup sliced Kalamata olives
1/4 cup reduced-fat feta cheese
3 tablespoons chopped fresh basil or 1 tablespoon dried basil leaves
2 tablespoons seasoned rice vinegar
Salt and pepper to taste

1 In medium pot, bring water to boil. Add couscous and follow directions on couscous container.

2 Transfer to large bowl and add all other ingredients, tossing carefully. Season to taste.

MAKES 6 (1-cup) servings
PREP TIME 10 minutes
COOK TIME 10 minutes

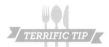
TERRIFIC TIP

I prefer the larger pearl or Israeli couscous, but any couscous may be used. Couscous is a type of coarsely ground semolina pasta, and can be found in the rice section of the grocery.

· · · · · · · · · · · · · · · · · ·

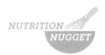
NUTRITION
NUGGET

Instead of couscous, wild rice may be used for gluten-free version.

NUTRITIONAL INFORMATION Calories 224, Calories from Fat 15%, Fat 4 g, Saturated Fat 1 g, Cholesterol 2 mg, Sodium 318 mg, Carbohydrates 40 g, Dietary Fiber 4 g, Total Sugars 3 g, Protein 7 g

DIABETIC EXCHANGES 2 1/2 starch, 1 vegetable, 1/2 fat

SOUTHWESTERN SWEET POTATO SALAD

Hard to beat this sensational and explosive combination of roasted sweet potatoes, crunchy corn, and black beans in a light jalapeño dressing.

6 cups peeled sweet potato chunks (about 2 1/2 pounds)
Salt and pepper to taste
3 tablespoons olive oil, divided
1/2 cup chopped red bell pepper
1/2 cup chopped red onion
2/3 cup frozen corn, thawed
2/3 cup black beans, drained and rinsed
1/4 cup chopped cilantro
3 tablespoons lime juice
1 teaspoon minced garlic
1 tablespoon jarred jalapeño slices

1 Preheat oven 425°F. Line baking pan with foil and coat with nonstick cooking spray.

2 On prepared pan, toss together sweet potatoes, salt and pepper and 1 tablespoon olive oil. Roast about 30 minutes or until potatoes are crisp. Cool.

3 In large bowl, combine sweet potatoes, red bell pepper, red onion, corn, black beans and cilantro.

4 In blender, puree lime juice, garlic, jalapeño and remaining 2 tablespoons oil. Toss with sweet potato mixture.

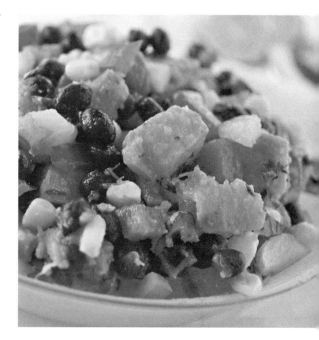

MAKES 12 (1/2-cup) servings
PREP TIME 20 minutes
COOK TIME 30 minutes

TERRIFIC TIP

Cook some burgers and take over this fabulous sweet potato salad for a fun dinner.

NUTRITION NUGGET

Their rich orange color lets you know sweet potatoes are rich in vitamin A and powerful anti-inflammatory antioxidants.

NUTRITIONAL INFORMATION Calories 113, Calories from fat 28%, Fat 4 g, Saturated Fat 0 g, Cholesterol 0 mg, Sodium 99 mg, Carbohydrate 19 g, Dietary Fiber 3 g, Total Sugars 4 g, Protein 2 g

DIABETIC EXCHANGES 1 1/2 starch, 1/2 fat

CHICKEN TOSTADAS

Don't let the long ingredient list intimidate you as this recipe has several parts: seasoned chicken, salsa, and avocado sauce. One of the best tasting tostadas you will EVER have!

- 1 tablespoon ground cumin
- 1 tablespoon chili powder
- 1 teaspoon garlic powder
- 1 teaspoon paprika
- Salt and pepper to taste
- 1 1/4 pounds chicken breasts, cubed
- 2 cups cherry tomato halves
- 1/4 cup finely chopped red onion
- 1 teaspoon minced garlic, divided
- 1/4 cup finely chopped cilantro
- 1 teaspoon olive oil
- 1 (15-ounce) can black beans, rinsed and drained
- 1 large avocado
- 3 tablespoons Greek nonfat plain yogurt
- 2 tablespoons lime juice
- 8 tostada shells
- 1/2 cup reduced-fat shredded Mexican-blend cheese

1. In small bowl, mix together cumin, chili powder, garlic powder, paprika, and season to taste. Toss chicken in seasonings. In large nonstick pan coated with nonstick cooking spray, cook chicken, stirring, until browned and cooked through; set aside.

2. In another bowl, combine tomatoes, red onion, 1/2 teaspoon garlic, 1/4 cup cilantro and olive oil. Season to taste; set aside. In another bowl, mix beans with remaining 1/2 teaspoon garlic; set aside.

3. In small bowl, mash avocado and add yogurt, lime juice and season to taste, mixing until smooth.

4. To assemble, spread guacamole on tostada and layer beans, tomato mixture, chicken and cheese.

MAKES 8 tostados

PREP TIME 20 minutes

COOK TIME 10 minutes

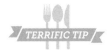

Prepare chicken, salsa and avocado mixtures in separate containers to put tostada together on your time frame. For a short cut, use seasoned rotisserie chicken and pick up salsa and guacamole.

• • • • • • • • • • • • • • • • • •

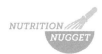

A serving of only 5 cherry tomatoes provide 15% of your daily recommended intake of vitamin A and 10% of vitamin C.

NUTRITIONAL INFORMATION Calories 297, Calories from Fat 37%, Fat 12 g, Saturated Fat 2 g, Cholesterol 50 mg, Sodium 405 mg, Carbohydrates 24 g, Dietary Fiber 7 g, Total Sugars 3 g, Protein 23 g

DIABETIC EXCHANGES 1 1/2 starch, 1 vegetable, 3 lean meat, 1/2 fat

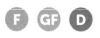

LEMON HERB SHRIMP

If your taste buds aren't working or your tummy aches, lemon flavors can be soothing. Serve this scrumptious shrimp and sauce with pasta and French bread.

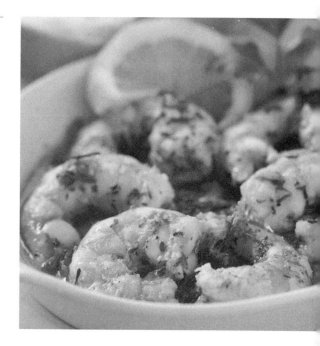

1/2 cup olive oil
2 teaspoons dried oregano leaves
2 teaspoons dried thyme leaves
1/2 cup chopped green onions
2 teaspoons grated lemon rind
1/4 cup lemon juice
Salt and pepper
2 pounds medium peeled shrimp, butterflied
 if possible

1 Combine all ingredients except shrimp in resealable plastic bag. Add shrimp, tossing to coat. Refrigerate one hour, time permitting.

2 Preheat oven 450°F. Place shrimp and marinade on foil lined baking pan.

3 Bake 10 minutes (depending on size of shrimp) or until shrimp is done and marinade is bubbling. Serve shrimp with sauce created from marinade.

MAKES **6–8 servings**
PREP TIME **5 minutes**
COOK TIME **10 minutes + time to marinate**

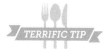

For lemon rind, finely grate or zest outside of lemon to get only lemon peel. Don't have lemon rind? Just leave it out.

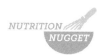

Fresh herbs can be substituted for dried herbs at a ratio of 3:1. In other words, 1 teaspoon of a dried herb= 1 tablespoon fresh.

NUTRITIONAL INFORMATION Calories 206, Calories from Fat 65%, Fat 15 g, Saturated Fat 2 g, Cholesterol 143 mg, Sodium 257 mg, Carbohydrates 3 g, Dietary Fiber 1 g, Total Sugars 0 g, Protein 16 g
DIABETIC EXCHANGES 2 lean meat, 2 fat

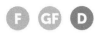

COMPANY CHICKEN

Fantastic and fabulous chicken dish. Serve with wild rice to enjoy the wonderful sauce.

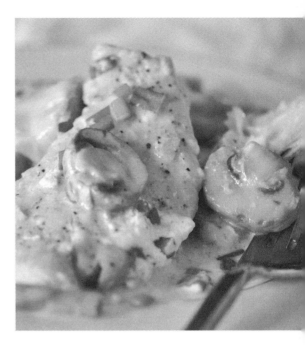

2 pounds boneless, skinless chicken breasts
Salt and pepper to taste
2 tablespoons butter
1/2 pound mushrooms, sliced
1/2 cup sherry or fat-free chicken broth
2 tablespoons lemon juice
1 (14-ounce) can quartered artichokes, drained
1 cup evaporated skimmed milk
1/2 cup chopped green onions
1/2 cup nonfat plain yogurt

1 Season chicken to taste. In large nonstick skillet coated with nonstick cooking spray, heat butter until melted. Brown chicken on both sides, 3–5 minutes each side. Add mushrooms, sherry, and lemon juice.

2 Bring to boil, reduce heat, cover, and cook, 20–30 minutes or until chicken is done.

3 Add artichokes and milk, stirring and cooking 5 more minutes. Stir in green onions and yogurt. Do not boil.

MAKES **6 servings**
PREP TIME **15 minutes**
COOK TIME **30 minutes**

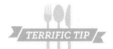
TERRIFIC TIP

Place chicken in one container and bring a zip-top bag of wild rice if making for someone. Freezes well.

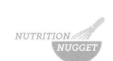
NUTRITION NUGGET

Artichokes are high in B vitamins, copper, and other minerals. B vitamins help convert carbohydrates into energy.

NUTRITIONAL INFORMATION Calories 287, Calories from Fat 19%, Fat 6 g, Saturated Fat 1 g, Cholesterol 90 mg, Sodium 330 mg, Carbohydrates 12 g, Dietary Fiber 1 g, Total Sugars 8 g, Protein 42 g
DIABETIC EXCHANGES 4 lean meat, 1/2 skim milk, 1 vegetable

LEMON FETA CHICKEN

I have more people tell me this is their favorite go-to quick chicken recipe because there are just a few ingredients to whip up this amazing chicken dish.

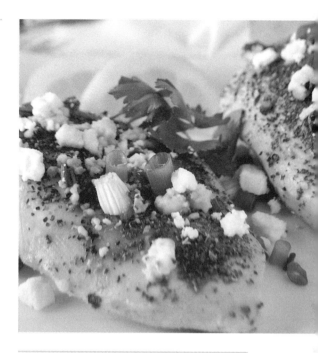

8 skinless, boneless chicken breasts
1/4 cup lemon juice, divided
1 tablespoon dried oregano leaves, divided
Pepper to taste
3 ounces crumbled reduced-fat feta cheese
3 tablespoons chopped green onions

1 Preheat oven 350°F. Coat 13×9×2-inch baking with nonstick cooking spray.

2 Place chicken in prepared baking dish, drizzle with half lemon juice. Sprinkle with half oregano and pepper. Top with cheese and green onions. Drizzle with remaining lemon juice and oregano.

3 Bake, covered, 45 minutes-1 hour, or until done.

MAKES **8 servings**
PREP TIME **5 minutes**
COOK TIME **45 minutes–1 hour**

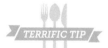

Don't like to cook but still want to bring someone a warm hearty dish? This simple recipe will be adored and it goes great with a side of angel hair pasta.

This diabetic-friendly dish is low on carbohydrates, lean in fat and high in satisfying flavorful protein.

NUTRITIONAL INFORMATION Calories 156, Calories from Fat 26%, Fat 4 g, Saturated Fat 2 g, Cholesterol 76 mg, Sodium 280 mg, Carbohydrates 1 g, Dietary Fiber 0 g, Total Sugars 0 g, Protein 26 g
DIABETIC EXCHANGES 3 1/2 lean meat

CHICKEN AND SAUSAGE JAMBALAYA

This is a quick and tasty one-dish meal. Jambalaya is a rice mixture combined with seasonings and is a great way to use leftover turkey or chicken.

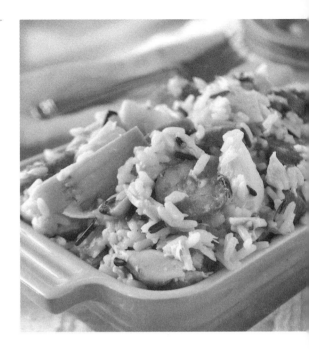

1 pound lower-fat turkey or chicken sausage, sliced
1 onion, chopped
1 pound fresh mushrooms, sliced
2 (6-ounce) packages long grain and wild rice mix
4 cups diced rotisserie chicken
1 (14-ounce) can artichoke hearts, quartered
1/2 cup chopped green onions

1 In large pot coated with nonstick cooking spray, brown sausage. Add onions and mushrooms, cooking until tender. Drain off excess grease.

2 Add wild rice, seasoning packet and water according to package directions to sausage mixture. Follow package directions for cooking time.

3 When done, toss with chicken and artichoke hearts; sprinkle with green onions.

MAKES **10 (1-cup) servings**
PREP TIME **10 minutes**
COOK TIME **30 minutes**

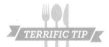
TERRIFIC TIP

Make easily with rotisserie chicken.

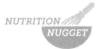
NUTRITION NUGGET

Artichokes are a naturally low-sodium, fat-free, low-calorie food, rich in healthy antioxidants and phytonutrients.

NUTRITIONAL INFORMATION Calories 332, Calories from Fat 23%, Fat 9 g, Saturated Fat 2 g, Cholesterol 93 mg, Sodium 828 mg, Carbohydrates 32 g, Dietary Fiber 2 g, Total Sugars 3 g, Protein 31 g

DIABETIC EXCHANGES 2 starch, 3 1/2 lean meat

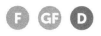

PULLED PORK

An easy, not-too-spicy pulled pork recipe that's made in a crock pot. Use for sandwiches, wraps, or with tortillas.

2 pounds pork tenderloin, cut into thirds
2 teaspoons cumin
1 1/2 cups salsa verde
1 onion, sliced
1 red bell pepper, cored and sliced

1 In 3 1/2–6 quart slow cooker, place pork tenderloin and add remaining ingredients.

2 Cook on LOW 6–8 or HIGH 4–5 hours or until tender. Shred with two forks.

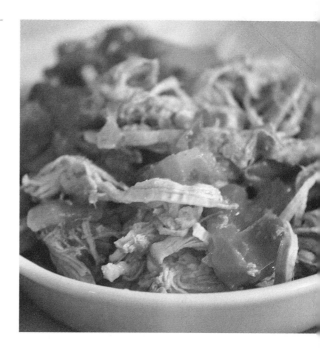

MAKES 8 (3/4-cup) servings
PREP TIME 5 minutes
COOK TIME 6–8 hours in crockpot

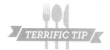

If serving with tortillas, top with avocado, onion, cheese and shredded cabbage. Salsa verde is a spicy green sauce made from tomatillos or green tomatoes (can be found in grocery).

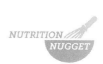

Ensure you are choosing the leanest cuts of meat by looking for those ending in "loin" or "round."

NUTRITIONAL INFORMATION Calories 134, Calories from Fat 21%, Fat 3 g, Saturated Fat 1 g, Cholesterol 60 mg, Sodium 190 mg, Carbohydrates 3 g, Dietary Fiber 0 g, Total Sugars 2 g, Protein 21 g

DIABETIC EXCHANGES 3 lean meat

F D

TURKEY PARMESAN MEATBALLS

Deliciously seasoned turkey meatballs topped with marinara and mozzarella make a yummy, lighter Italian dish. Serve with pasta, couscous or alone.

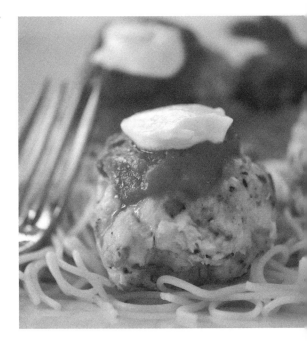

1 1/4 pounds ground white meat turkey
1/2 cup Italian bread crumbs
1/2 cup chopped onion
2 teaspoons dried basil leaves
2 teaspoons dried oregano leaves
2 teaspoons minced garlic
2 egg whites, beaten
1/4 cup grated Parmesan cheese
Salt and black pepper to taste
2 cups healthy marinara sauce
3-ounces fresh mozzarella cheese

1 Preheat oven 400°F. Line baking pan with foil and coat with nonstick cooking spray.

2 In large bowl, mix together turkey, bread crumbs, onion, basil, oregano, garlic, egg whites, Parmesan cheese and season to taste. With moistened hands, shape into balls a little larger than golf ball. Place on prepared pan. Bake 15–20 minutes or until done.

3 Remove meatballs from oven, spoon marinara sauce on top of each meatball, and top each with small piece mozzarella cheese. Bake approximately another 3–5 minutes or until cheese is melted.

MAKES 6 (3-meatball) servings
PREP TIME 20 minutes
COOK TIME 25 minutes

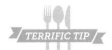
TERRIFIC TIP

Look for "healthy" marinara sauce in the grocery, for a low-sodium, low-sugar option. These individual meatballs make it easy to serve as an appetizer.

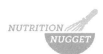
NUTRITION NUGGET

You can serve as a snack or small plate since the meatballs are served individually.

NUTRITIONAL INFORMATION Calories 256, Calories from Fat 23%, Fat 7 g, Saturated Fat 2 g, Cholesterol 52 mg, Sodium 596 mg, Carbohydrates 18 g, Dietary Fiber 3 g, Total Sugars 8 g, Protein 32 g
DIABETIC EXCHANGES 1 starch, 3 1/2 lean meat

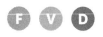

WHITE SPINACH AND ARTICHOKE PIZZA

A light creamy white sauce topped with spinach, artichokes, sun-dried tomatoes, Italian seasoning and cheese turns pizza into a delectable and comforting meal.

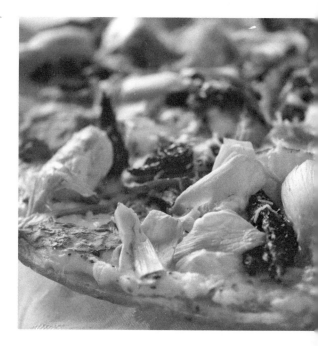

1 cup skim milk
3 tablespoons all-purpose flour
1/2 teaspoon minced garlic
Salt and pepper to taste
1 (12-inch) thin pizza crust
1 cup coarsely chopped baby spinach
Half small red onion, thinly sliced and halved
1 (14-ounce) can quartered artichokes, drained
3 tablespoons sun-dried tomatoes
1 teaspoon dried basil leaves
1 teaspoon dried oregano leaves
1 cup shredded part-skim mozzarella cheese

MAKES **8 servings**
PREP TIME **10 minutes**
COOK TIME **10 minutes**

1 Preheat oven 425°F.

2 In small nonstick pot, combine milk and flour over medium heat, stirring until thickened. Add garlic and season to taste.

3 Spread white sauce over crust. Top with spinach, onion, artichokes and sun-dried tomatoes. Sprinkle with basil, oregano, and mozzarella cheese.

4 Bake 10 minutes or until crust is golden brown and cheese is melted.

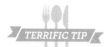
TERRIFIC TIP

Instead of picking up a frozen pizza, make your own for the freezer. Don't cook before freezing. Fresh tomatoes may be substituted for sun-dried tomatoes.

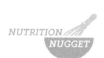
NUTRITION NUGGET

You know spinach is chocked full of nutrition by it's vibrant rich green color—concentrated in phytonutrients and flavonoids, offering healthy antioxidant protection.

NUTRITIONAL INFORMATION Calories 169, Calories from Fat 23%, Fat 4 g, Saturated Fat 2 g, Cholesterol 10 mg, Sodium 379 mg, Carbohydrates 23 g, Dietary Fiber 1 g, Total Sugars 3 g, Protein 10 g
DIABETIC EXCHANGES **1 1/2 starch, 1 lean meat**

HEALTHY EATING

Simple, nutritious time-efficient recipes with everyday ingredients for an overall healthier lifestyle.

. . . .

Do I have to follow a special diet?

Is it okay to eat raw fruits and vegetables?

Are there any foods that decrease my risk of cancer?

What is the most important food to decrease for healthy living?

What about carcinogens—a cancer producing substance?

. . . .

Once your treatments are over, you will hopefully start to feel better and will be eager to try new foods. Your taste buds are alert again and ready to be stimulated. You do not have to worry about your blood count being low or your mouth being sore. Hopefully, your bowel habits have normalized. It is fine to eat raw fruits and vegetables.

Salt-cured and pickled foods contain natural carcinogens that may increase your risk of developing stomach and esophageal cancers. Nitrates and nitrites, used to preserve meats, can enhance the formation of nitrosoamine, another carcinogen. Smoked foods can absorb carcinogens out of the smoke.

Please do not forget smoking is the very worst carcinogen around. Smoking is responsible for lung, bladder, esophageal, and head and neck cancer. Eat healthy, and **PLEASE DO NOT SMOKE**.

Healthy foods, such as whole grains, legumes, fruits and vegetables, will decrease your risk of cancer. These foods all contain dietary fiber, which is thought to protect against colon cancer.

Diets high in fruits and vegetables are believed to protect against bladder, prostate, stomach, esophageal, and lung cancer. Cruciferous vegetables (kale, cauliflower,

broccoli) may also reduce your risk of cancer. Foods rich in vitamin C can protect against cancers of the mouth, esophagus, pancreas, and stomach.

Vitamins A and E may help protect against certain cancers by acting as antioxidants, and in the case of vitamin E, by inhibiting the conversion of nitrites into nitrosamines. Green tea may protect against some cancers by stimulating the activity of antioxidants and detoxifying enzymes. Also note that a diet that reduces your risk of developing cancer can also reduce your risk of developing heart disease. It can also decrease your risk of developing diverticulitis and irritable bowel syndrome, both of which have been linked to a diet low in fiber.

There are more studies on fat than on any other dietary risk factor. There is good evidence that fat increases your risk of developing cancer, especially cancer of the prostate, colon, breast, ovary, endometrium, and pancreas.

The 2015–2020 Dietary Guidelines for Americans recommend saturated fat intake should be limited to less than 10 percent of calories per day and they should be replaced with unsaturated fats, while keeping total dietary fats within the age-appropriate

AMDR (Acceptable Macronutrient Distribution Ranges). Strategies to lower saturated fat intake include:

- Choose packaged foods lower in saturated fats by reading food labels.
- Choose lower fat milk (such as skim or low-fat milk rather than 2% or whole milk)
- Replace ice cream with sherbet or frozen yogurt or use low-fat products.
- Choose low fat cheese.
- Choose meat with "loin" or "round" in the name—for example: ground sirloin.
- Eat skinless chicken or turkey breasts.
- Replace meat with beans, fish or chicken.
- Prepare foods using oils high in poly-unsaturated and monounsaturated fats instead of solid fats high in saturated fat.
- Use oil-based condiments instead of those made with solid fats (such as butter, stick margarine, cream cheese).

The 2015–2020 Dietary Guidelines for Americans recommend trans fat intake should be as low as possible. Research shows that increased intake of trans fats is linked to increased risk of cardiovascular disease.

- Avoid synthetic or artificial trans fatty acids by limiting intake of partially hydrogenated oils found in margarine and many processed foods.
- Substitute croissants and breakfast bars with bagels, English muffins, whole grain bread, pita bread or corn tortillas.
- Natural trans fatty acids are found in dairy and meat in small quantities. Do not remove these foods from the diet, instead choose low-fat dairy and lean meats to reduce trans fat intake.
- Be conscious of your choice of food.

Remember you do not have to deprive yourself forever of the foods you love. If you over do it one day, make allowances the next day or two. The method of healthy eating Monday through Friday and splurging on the weekends sometimes works well for people. It is important that you find the balance of what works best for you. Your goal is a long term healthy lifestyle. With all these tasty recipes, you will find that your diet will not be different than the next person as it is the approach in preparation of these recipes that has changed. Enjoy eating and staying healthy.

There is not one food or food group that is most important to survivorship. A healthy balanced diet within moderation, and according to the Dietary Guidelines, is the best recommendation for food intake.

KEY RECOMMENDATIONS OF HEALTHY EATING

The 2015–2020 Dietary Guidelines for Americans recommends that you consume:

- Food and beverage within your appropriate calorie range.
- A variety of colorful vegetables (green, red, orange, yellow, purple, etc.)
- Fruit, especially whole fruit.
- Fat-free or low-fat dairy (milk, cheese, yogurt)
- A variety of lean protein (seafood, poultry, lean meat, eggs, legumes, nuts and seeds)
- Unsaturated oils.
- Less than 10 percent of calories per day from added sugars, and the same for saturated fat.
- Less than 2,300 milligrams (mg) per day of sodium.
- Alcohol in moderation, if at all.

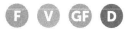

OATMEAL BANANA PANCAKES

Whip up these easy, great morning pancakes with an added dose of "good for you" ingredients. Keep in your freezer to pull out.

2 cups old-fashioned oatmeal
2 cups water
1 banana, cut into chunks
2 tablespoons maple syrup or honey
Dash salt
1 teaspoon vanilla extract

1. In blender or food processor, add all ingredients; blend until smooth. Let stand 5 minutes until batter thickens.

2. In nonstick skillet coasted with nonstick cooking spray, pour about 1/4–1/3 cup batter into pan and cook 2–3 minutes on each side or until golden brown.

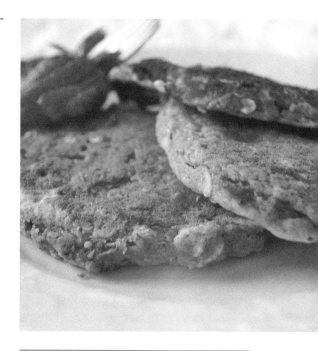

MAKES 16 pancakes
PREP TIME 5 minutes
COOK TIME 10 minutes

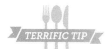

Sometimes I add a little cinnamon. These pancakes freeze great.

Oats are an excellent source of soluble fiber which helps keep you feeling full longer, as well as stabilizing blood sugar.

NUTRITIONAL INFORMATION Calories 51, Calories from Fat 13%, Fat 1 g, Saturated Fat 0 g, Cholesterol 0 mg, Sodium 9 mg, Carbohydrates 10 g, Dietary Fiber 1 g, Total Sugars 3 g, Protein 1 g

DIABETIC EXCHANGES 1/2 starch

SPINACH SALAD WITH STRAWBERRIES

With its subtly sweet vinaigrette paired with fresh fruit, this salad has been one of my most popular salads for years.

3 tablespoons raspberry wine vinegar
3 tablespoons raspberry jam
1/4 cup canola oil
8 cups fresh baby spinach (or mixed greens)
1 pint strawberries, sliced
3 kiwis, peeled and sliced
2 teaspoons sesame seeds

1 Combine vinegar and jam in food processor or blender. Add oil in thin stream, blending well; set aside.

2 Carefully toss fresh spinach, strawberries, kiwis and sesame seeds with vinaigrette. Serve immediately.

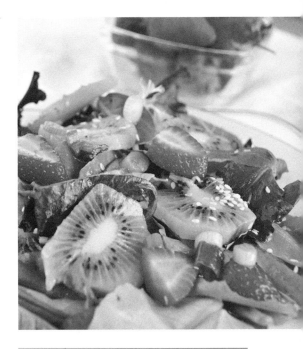

MAKES 8 (1 1/4-cup) servings
PREP TIME 10 minutes

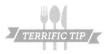
TERRIFIC TIP

Raspberries may be substituted for strawberries and use any combination of mixed greens. You can buy vinaigrette instead of making one also.

DOC'S NOTE

Berries are little jewels packed with fiber and antioxidants that help slow the aging process from the inside out. Did you know sesame seeds are loaded with calcium?

NUTRITIONAL INFORMATION Calories 122, Calories from Fat 55%, Fat 8 g, Saturated Fat 1 g, Cholesterol 0 mg, Sodium 25 mg, Carbohydrates 13 g, Dietary Fiber 2 g, Total Sugars 9 g, Protein 2 g

DIABETIC EXCHANGES 1 fruit, 1 1/2 fat

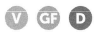

WATERMELON AND TOMATO SALAD

This combination of cool crisp watermelon, juicy tomatoes, and fresh basil with balsamic vinegar creates an extraordinary and invigorating light salad.

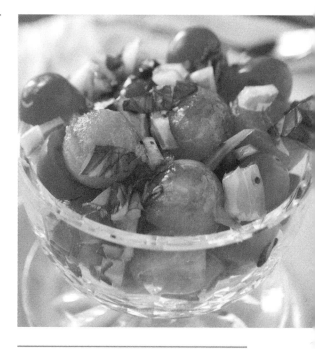

4 cups scooped out watermelon balls or chunks
1/2 cup chopped red onion
1 pint cherry tomatoes, halved
2 tablespoons fresh chopped basil
1 tablespoon olive oil
2 tablespoons balsamic vinegar
Salt to taste

1 In bowl, combine watermelon, onion, tomatoes and basil.

2 Whisk together oil and vinegar, toss with salad. Season to taste. Serve immediately or that day.

MAKES 10 (1/2 cup) servings
PREP TIME 15 minutes

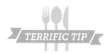

Perfect way to use leftover watermelon that sits in the refrigerator.

· · · · · · · · · · · · · · · ·

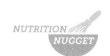

Although water accounts for over 90% of watermelon's weight, it is also a rich source of potassium, and vitamins A and C.

NUTRITIONAL INFORMATION Calories 46, Calories from Fat 29%, Fat 2 g, Saturated Fat 0 g, Cholesterol 0 mg, Sodium 6 mg, Carbohydrates 8 g, Dietary Fiber 1 g, Total Sugars 6 g, Protein 1 g

DIABETIC EXCHANGES 1/2 fruit, 1/2 fat

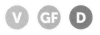

CAESAR SALAD

Try my healthier version of this classic favorite.

1 large head romaine lettuce, torn into pieces
  (about 8 cups)
1/4 cup grated Parmesan cheese
1/2 cup plain nonfat Greek yogurt
1/2 teaspoon minced garlic
2 tablespoons lemon juice
1 teaspoon vinegar
1 teaspoon Worcestershire sauce
1 teaspoon Dijon mustard
1 tablespoon sesame seeds

1. In large bowl, combine lettuce and cheese.

2. In small bowl, whisk together remaining ingredients. Toss with lettuce.

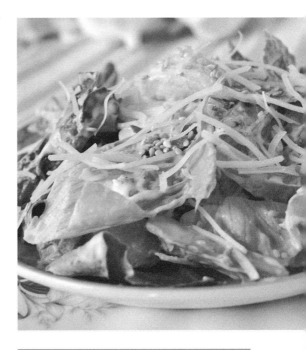

MAKES 4 heaping (1-cup) servings
PREP TIME 5 minutes

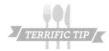

Use this dressing over other salads and always think about adding additional veggies to your salad.

. . . .

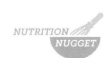

The greener or more vibrant the color of the lettuce, the more nutrition.

NUTRITIONAL INFORMATION Calories 73, Calories from Fat 38%, Fat 3 g, Saturated Fat 1 g, Cholesterol 4 mg, Sodium 135 mg, Carbohydrates 6 g, Dietary Fiber 2 g, Total Sugars 3 g, Protein 6 g

DIABETIC EXCHANGES 1 vegetable, 1/2 lean meat

(V) (GF)

BRUSSELS SPROUTS, TOMATO, AND FETA SALAD

Roasting Brussels Sprouts brings out the sweetness combined with tomatoes and feta, you get a remarkable salad.

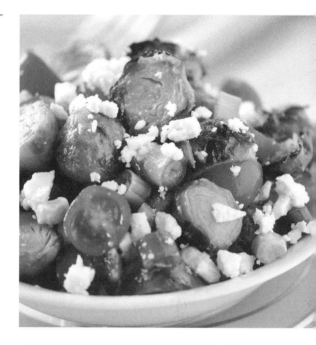

1 1/4 pounds Brussels sprouts
2 teaspoons plus 3 tablespoons olive oil, divided
1/4 cup white balsamic vinegar
1 tablespoon Dijon mustard
Salt and pepper to taste
1 cup grape or cherry tomatoes, halved
3 tablespoons chopped green onions
1/4 cup reduced-fat feta cheese

1 Preheat oven 450°F. Line baking pan with foil and coat with nonstick cooking spray.

2 Remove outer discolored leaves from Brussels sprouts and cut in half. Place on prepared pan and drizzle with 2 teaspoons oil, tossing. Bake 20–25 minutes or until tender. Cool.

3 In small bowl, whisk together vinegar, Dijon, remaining 3 tablespoons oil, and season to taste.

4 In bowl, combine Brussels sprouts, tomatoes, green onions, and feta; toss with vinaigrette. Serve at room temperature or chilled.

MAKES 5 (1-cup) servings
PREP TIME 15 minutes
COOK TIME 25 minutes

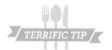
TERRIFIC TIP

If you don't have white balsamic vinegar, any vinegar may be used.

· · · · · · · · · · · · · · · ·

DOC'S NOTE

Brussels sprouts have DNA protective and cancer preventative benefits.

NUTRITIONAL INFORMATION Calories 176, Calories from Fat 54%, Fat 12 g, Saturated Fat 2 g, Cholesterol 2 mg, Sodium 193 mg, Carbohydrates 16 g, Dietary Fiber 5 g, Total Sugars 7 g, Protein 6 g

DIABETIC EXCHANGES 3 vegetable, 2 1/2 fat

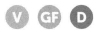

ASIAN SLAW
WITH GINGER-PEANUT VINAIGRETTE

Slaw, carrots, red pepper, edamame and peanuts tossed with Ginger-Peanut Vinaigrette create a quick-fix, easy slaw bursting with flavor.

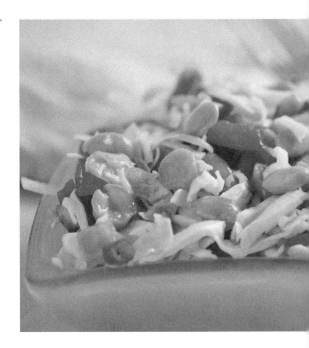

4 cups prepared shredded coleslaw
1/2 cup finely chopped or shredded carrots
1 red pepper, thinly sliced into 1-inch pieces
1/2 cup shelled edamame
1/2 cup chopped green onions
1/3 cup salted peanuts

1 In large bowl, combine coleslaw, carrots, red pepper, edamame, green onions, and peanuts.

2 Toss slaw with Ginger-Peanut Vinaigrette. Let sit at least 10 minutes before serving. Refrigerate.

MAKES 10 (1/2 cup) servings

PREP TIME 15 minutes

GINGER-PEANUT VINAIGRETTE

1/4 cup honey
2 tablespoons canola oil
1/4 cup seasoned rice vinegar
1 tablespoon low-sodium soy sauce
1 tablespoon peanut butter
1 tablespoon minced fresh ginger
1/2 teaspoon minced garlic

1 In small bowl, whisk together vinaigrette ingredients until peanut butter is mixed in.

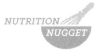

TERRIFIC TIP

Try using Angel Hair Cole Slaw for its nice delicate, finely shredded cabbage.

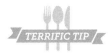

NUTRITION NUGGET

I keep frozen, shelled edamame in my freezer to pop out and thaw, adding a quick protein crunch and zing to recipes.

NUTRITIONAL INFORMATION Calories 120, Calories from Fat 47%, Fat 7 g, Saturated Fat 1 g, Cholesterol 0 mg, Sodium 152 mg, Carbohydrates 13 g, Dietary Fiber 2 g, Total Sugars 11 g, Protein 3 g

DIABETIC EXCHANGES 1 vegetable, 1 other carbohydrate, 1 1/2 fat

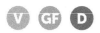

GREAT GARDEN SALAD

Color equals nutrition and this salad is overflowing with flavor, color and garden fresh favorites.

1 1/2 cups fresh or frozen corn
1 cup chopped tomatoes
1 cup chopped peeled cucumber
1/3 cup shelled edamame, cooked according to directions and drained
1/2 cup chopped red onion
1/3 cup chopped avocado
2 tablespoons lime juice
1 tablespoon olive oil
Salt and pepper to taste

1 In bowl, combine corn, tomatoes, cucumber, edamame, red onion, and avocado.

2 In small bowl, whisk together lime juice and oil. Toss with corn mixture and season to taste.

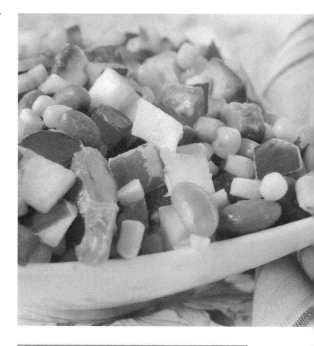

MAKES 6 (2/3-cup) servings
PREP TIME 10 minutes

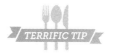

TERRIFIC TIP

Look for frozen shelled edamame in the frozen vegetable section.

· · · · · · · · · · · · · · · · ·

DOC'S NOTE

Tomatoes are one of the best sources of lycopene, a powerful antioxidant helping reduce the risk for heart disease and some cancers.

NUTRITIONAL INFORMATION Calories 92, Calories from fat 42%, Fat 4 g, Saturated Fat 1 g, Cholesterol 0 mg, Sodium 9 mg, Carbohydrate 12 g, Dietary Fiber 3 g, Total Sugars 3 g, Protein 3 g
DIABETIC EXCHANGES 1/2 starch, 1 vegetable, 1/2 fat

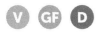

KALE SALAD
WITH FRUITY VINAIGRETTE

Don't turn up your nose to kale until you taste this simple, captivating, fantastic salad.

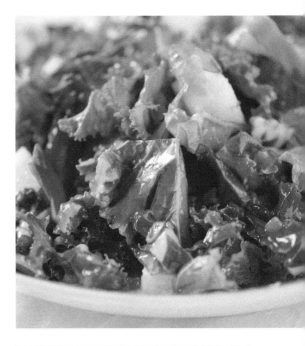

8 cups chopped kale, center ribs and stems removed
1 cup shredded red cabbage
1 apple, nectarine or fruit of choice, chopped
1/3 cup chopped pecans, toasted

1 In large bowl, toss together kale, cabbage, fruit and pecans.

2 Toss salad with Fruity Vinaigrette.

FRUITY VINAIGRETTE

3 tablespoons olive oil
2 tablespoons apple cider vinegar
1/4 cup apricot preserves
2 tablespoons lemon juice
1 teaspoon Dijon mustard

1 In small bowl, whisk together all vinaigrette ingredients.

MAKES 8 servings
PREP TIME 10 minutes

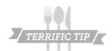

Kale is all the rage but kale is easy to use as you can find pre-chopped kale in bags at the grocery for short-cut.

· · · · · · · · · · · · · · · · · ·

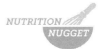

Use heart-healthy olive oil for the vinaigrette; although calorie dense, a little olive oil goes a long way, working to block enzymes involved in inflammation—acting like ibuprofen.

NUTRITIONAL INFORMATION Calories 145, Calories from Fat 52%, Fat 9 g, Saturated Fat 1 g, Cholesterol 0 mg, Sodium 44 mg, Carbohydrates 16 g, Dietary Fiber 2 g, Total Sugars 7 g, Protein 3 g
DIABETIC EXCHANGES 1/2 fruit, 2 vegetable, 2 fat

ROASTED BUTTERNUT SQUASH, KALE, AND CRANBERRY COUSCOUS

Naturally sweet butternut squash, crunchy kale, and tart cranberries mix with couscous for a dynamic recipe. Serve hot, room temperature, or chilled.

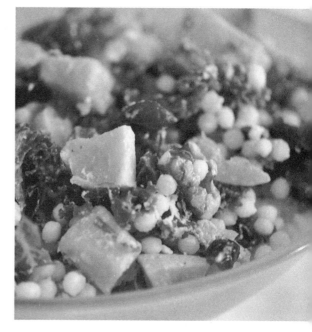

4 cups cubed butternut squash

Salt and pepper to taste

1 cup pearl couscous, cooked in water according to package instructions

2 cups coarsely chopped kale leaves

3 tablespoons dried cranberries

1/4 cup chopped walnuts, toasted

2 ounces crumbled goat cheese, optional

1 Preheat oven 425°F. Line baking pan with foil and coat with nonstick cooking spray

2 Arrange squash on prepared pan; season to taste. Coat with nonstick cooking spray. Bake 15 minutes, stir, and continue baking 10-15 minutes or until tender. Remove from oven.

3 In a large bowl, combine cooked squash, cooked couscous, kale, cranberries, walnuts, and goat cheese, if desired. Toss with Orange Vinaigrette.

ORANGE VINAIGRETTE

2 tablespoons apple cider vinegar

1 tablespoon olive oil

3 tablespoons orange juice

1 In small bowl, whisk together all vinaigrette ingredients.

MAKES 6 (1-cup) servings

PREP TIME 15 minutes

COOK TIME 30 minutes

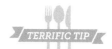

With pre-cut butternut squash, chopped kale, and quick cooking couscous, this is a speedy salad. Any type of couscous can be used.

. . . .

You are eating with nutrition with this recipe—each color providing important protective vitamins and nutrients.

NUTRITIONAL INFORMATION Calories 230, Calories from Fat 22%, Fat 6 g, Saturated Fat 1 g, Cholesterol 0 mg, Sodium 16 mg, Carbohydrates 40 g, Dietary Fiber 4 g, Total Sugars 5 g, Protein 6 g

DIABETIC EXCHANGES 2 1/2 starch, 1 fat

V GF D

QUINOA SALAD
WITH THAI VINAIGRETTE

How could such an antioxidant packed salad be so simple to make and so wonderful to eat? The Thai Vinaigrette perfectly complements the fresh crunchy ingredients and hearty quinoa.

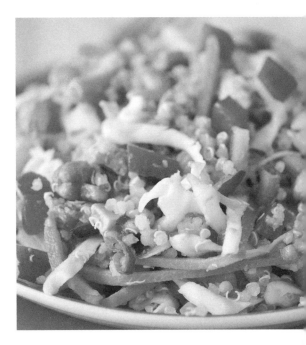

3/4 cup uncooked quinoa
2 cups shredded red cabbage
1 red bell pepper, cored and chopped
2/3 cup chopped red onion
1 cup shredded carrot
1 bunch green onions, chopped
1/2 cup cashew halves

1 Prepare quinoa according to package directions. When done, fluff with fork.

2 In large bowl, combine cooked quinoa with remaining ingredients. Toss with Thai Vinaigrette and serve.

THAI VINAIGRETTE
Peanut butter, ginger, soy sauce, and honey with a touch of sesame oil create a winner!

3 tablespoons peanut butter
2 teaspoon grated fresh ginger
3 tablespoons low-sodium soy sauce
1 tablespoon honey
1 tablespoon red wine vinegar
1 teaspoon sesame oil
1 teaspoon olive oil

1 In small bowl, whisk together all vinaigrette ingredients. Add water to thin, if needed.

MAKES 8 (1 cup) servings
PREP TIME 15 minutes
COOK TIME 15 minutes

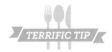

Can also serve as a side salad. Add Rotisserie chicken, grilled shrimp or whatever protein you want for a heartier version.

. . . .

Although usually considered a whole grain, quinoa is actually a seed or legume that contains all 9 essential amino acids, making it a complete protein, great for vegetarians.

NUTRITIONAL INFORMATION Calories 193, Calories from Fat 47%, Fat 10 g, Saturated Fat 2 g, Cholesterol 0 mg, Sodium 208 mg, Carbohydrates 23 g, Dietary Fiber 3 g, Total Sugars 8 g, Protein 7 g

DIABETIC EXCHANGES 1 1/2 starch, 1 fat, 1 vegetable

ASIAN CHICKEN PASTA SALAD

Simple and effortless wonderful salad with Asian-infused flavor.

12 ounces bow tie pasta
4 cups shredded skinless chicken breasts (rotisserie chicken)
4 cups packed baby spinach
1 bunch green onions, chopped
1 (11-ounce) can mandarin oranges, drained and reserve 3 tablespoons juice
1/2 cup shelled edamame
1/3 cup sliced almonds, toasted

1 Prepare pasta according to package directions: drain and set aside.

2 Toss chicken with 1/2 cup Asian Vinaigrette; set aside.

3 In large bowl, combine spinach, green onions, mandarin oranges, and edamame. Add chicken.

4 Toss with remaining Asian Vinaigrette. Gently mix in almonds and serve immediately.

ASIAN VINAIGRETTE

1/4 cup low-sodium soy sauce
1/4 cup red wine vinegar
3 tablespoons reserved mandarin orange juice
2 tablespoons sesame or canola oil
2 tablespoons sesame seeds, toasted
2 teaspoons sugar

1 In small bowl, whisk together all vinaigrette ingredients.

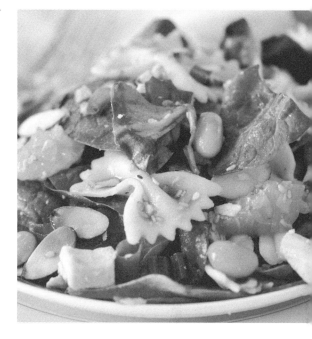

MAKES 12 (1 cup) servings
PREP TIME 15 minutes
COOK TIME 15 minutes

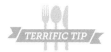

TERRIFIC TIP

Rotisserie chicken is a lean, protein-rich time-saver. Look for toasted sesame seeds in the Asian or spice section.

. . . .

NUTRITION NUGGET

Along with fiber, spinach is rich in antioxidants providing excellent anti-inflammatory benefits. Sesame seeds are packed with calcium.

NUTRITIONAL INFORMATION Calories 253, Calories from Fat 25%, Fat 7 g, Saturated Fat 1 g, Cholesterol 42 mg, Sodium 307 mg, Carbohydrates 28 g, Dietary Fiber 3 g, Total Sugars 6 g, Protein 20 g

DIABETIC EXCHANGES 2 starch, 2 lean meat

SHRIMP, CORN, AND SWEET POTATO SOUP

The unique combination of naturally sweet and nutritious sweet potatoes with shrimp and corn makes a rich, bold flavored one-pot meal.

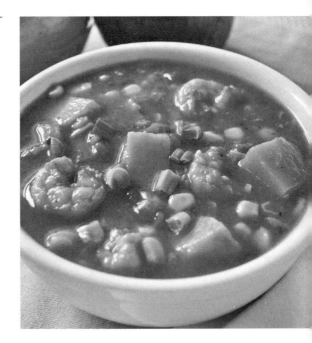

1 red onion, chopped
1/2 cup chopped celery
1/2 teaspoon minced garlic
1 green bell pepper, chopped
2 cups peeled, diced sweet potatoes
1 (16-ounce) bag frozen corn
1 (14 3/4-ounce) can cream-style corn
1 (10-ounce) can chopped tomatoes and green chilies
1 (6-ounce) can low-sodium tomato paste
4 cups fat-free, low-sodium chicken broth
1 1/2 pounds peeled medium shrimp
Salt and pepper to taste
1/2 cup chopped green onions

1   In large nonstick pot coated with nonstick cooking spray, sauté onion, celery, garlic, and green pepper over medium heat 5–7 minutes or until tender.

2   Add sweet potatoes, corn, cream-style corn, tomatoes and green chilies, tomato paste, and broth and bring mixture to a boil.

3   Add shrimp and cook about 10 minutes or until shrimp is done. Season to taste. Sprinkle with green onions before serving.

MAKES 12 (1 cup) servings
PREP TIME 15 minutes
COOK TIME 25 minutes

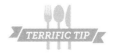
TERRIFIC TIP

For a short cut, look at the grocery for a container of pre-chopped seasonings. Freeze in containers.

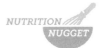
NUTRITION NUGGET

Their rich orange color lets you know sweet potatoes are rich in vitamin A and powerful anti-inflammatory antioxidants.

NUTRITIONAL INFORMATION Calories 149, Calories from Fat 11%, Fat 1 g, Saturated Fat 0 g, Cholesterol 84 mg, Sodium 344 mg, Carbohydrates 24 g, Dietary Fiber 4 g, Total Sugars 6 g, Protein 13 g
DIABETIC EXCHANGES 1 1/2 starch, 1 very lean meat

GF D

CHICKEN LETTUCE WRAPS

Fast and fantastic, if you've never had lettuce wraps, you're in for a treat as this light meal comes together easily with rotisserie chicken, bell pepper, edamame and sweet mango with a super sauce.

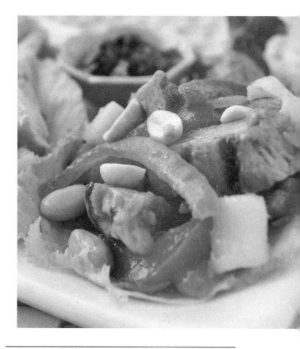

1 onion, halved and thinly sliced
1 red bell pepper, cored and thinly sliced
1 teaspoon minced garlic
1 1/2 teaspoons grated fresh ginger
1/2 cup shelled edamame
1 tablespoon low-sodium soy sauce
3 tablespoons seasoned rice vinegar
1 teaspoon cornstarch, mixed with 1 tablespoon water
2 cups chopped skinless rotisserie chicken breast
1 cup chopped mango
2 tablespoons chopped peanuts
Boston or red tip lettuce leaves

1. In large nonstick skillet, sauté onion and bell pepper, cooking until onion is almost tender, about 5 minutes. Add garlic, ginger, and edamame; stirring, about 1 minute.

2. Stir in soy sauce, vinegar, and cornstarch mixture, heating mixture until thickens. Remove from heat and add chicken, mango and peanuts. Spoon mixture onto lettuce and wrap.

MAKES 8 (1/2-cup filling) wraps
PREP TIME 15 minutes
COOK TIME 7 minutes

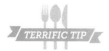
TERRIFIC TIP

I serve my wraps with hoisin sauce. For fresh ginger, 1/2 teaspoon ground ginger may be used. I like adding fruit such as mango, but it can be omitted, if desired.

· · · · · · · · · · · · · · · · ·

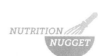
NUTRITION NUGGET

Soybeans, or edamame, are a good source of fiber—1 cup cooked provides over 40% of your daily recommended intake—and are an excellent source of plant protein, containing all essential amino acids.

NUTRITIONAL INFORMATION Calories 104, Calories from Fat 24%, Fat 3 g, Saturated Fat 0 g, Cholesterol 32 mg, Sodium 172 mg, Carbohydrates 8 g, Dietary Fiber 2 g, Total Sugars 5 g, Protein 13 g

DIABETIC EXCHANGES 1/2 other carbohydrate, 1 1/2 lean meat

SALSA CHICKEN

Whip up this quick Mexican dish with chicken and four ingredients. Serve over yellow rice to enjoy the tasty southwestern sauce.

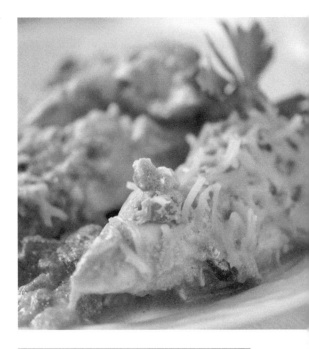

2 cups salsa
1 cup nonfat sour cream
1 (1-ounce) package low-sodium taco seasoning
1 1/2 pounds boneless, skinless chicken breast tenders
1/2 cup reduced-fat sharp Cheddar cheese
Cilantro or green onions, chopped, optional

1 Preheat oven 350°F. Coat oblong glass baking dish with nonstick cooking spray.

2 In bowl, mix together salsa, sour cream, and taco seasoning.

3 Place chicken into prepared dish. Pour sauce over chicken and bake 45 minutes or until chicken is tender. Sprinkle with cheese and cilantro or green onions, if desired.

MAKES 6 servings
PREP TIME 5 minutes
COOK TIME 45 minutes

TERRIFIC TIP

A jar of salsa works fine but try using fresh salsa found in the grocery.

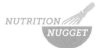

NUTRITION NUGGET

Did you know that 1/2 cup of salsa equals one serving of vegetables? All the more reason to dig in!

NUTRITIONAL INFORMATION Calories 238, Calories from Fat 19%, Fat 5 g, Saturated Fat 2 g, Cholesterol 85 mg, Sodium 776 mg, Carbohydrates 15 g, Dietary Fiber 0 g, Total Sugars 5 g, Protein 29 g
DIABETIC EXCHANGES 1 other carbohydrate, 3 lean meat

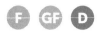

HONEY CHICKEN AND BROCCOLI STIR-FRY

Bored with chicken? Try this quick chicken stir-fry that effortlessly perks up chicken and veggies.

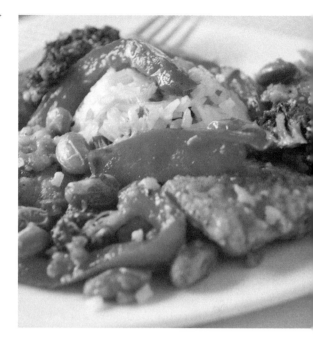

2 cups broccoli florets
1 red bell pepper, cored and thinly sliced
1 teaspoon minced garlic
2 egg whites plus 1 tablespoon water
1/3 cup cornstarch
3 tablespoons olive oil
1 1/2 pounds boneless, skinless, chicken breasts,
  cut in chunks or strips
1 cup edamame
1/4 cup honey
1-2 tablespoons low-sodium soy sauce
Salt and pepper to taste

1 In large nonstick pan coated with nonstick cooking spray, add broccoli, red bell pepper and garlic, sauté about 5 minutes; set aside.

2 In two shallow bowls, put egg whites with water and in the other, cornstarch. In same pan, heat olive oil. When pan is hot, dip chicken pieces in egg whites and then lightly dredge in cornstarch. Add to pan and brown 2–3 minutes, then turn and continue cooking and stirring until chicken is browned and done, 5–7 minutes.

3 Add reserved broccoli mixture and edamame to pan with chicken. Add honey and soy sauce, stirring until chicken is thoroughly coated and mixture heated. Season to taste.

MAKES 6 (1-cup) servings
PREP TIME 20 minutes
COOK TIME 20 minutes

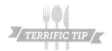

TERRIFIC TIP

Serve with rice tossed with green onions. To turn into a Beef and Broccoli Stir Fry, use thinly sliced flank steak for the chicken. I use edamame for an added nutritional boost but you can leave it out.

· · · · · · · · · · · · · · · ·

NUTRITION NUGGET

Did you know that broccoli is actually a significant source of highly absorbable calcium and red pepper has more vitamin C than an orange?

NUTRITIONAL INFORMATION Calories 317, Calories from Fat 32%, Fat 11 g, Saturated Fat 2 g, Cholesterol 73 mg, Sodium 229 mg, Carbohydrates 24 g, Dietary Fiber 3 g, Total Sugars 14 g, Protein 30 g

DIABETIC EXCHANGES 1 vegetable, 1 1/2 other carbohydrate, 3 1/2 lean meat

CHICKEN, RED PEPPER, SPINACH AND WHITE BEAN PIZZA

An exceptional tasty pizza with a hearty combination of chicken, spinach, and beans.

1 (12-inch) thin pizza crust
2 teaspoons olive oil
1 medium red bell pepper, cored and thinly sliced
1/2 cup chopped red onion
1 teaspoon minced garlic
2 cups chopped baby spinach
1 teaspoon dried oregano leaves
1 cup chopped cooked chicken breast
1/2 cup white navy beans, drained and rinsed
1 cup shredded part-skim mozzarella cheese

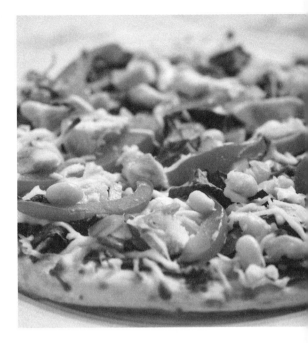

1. Preheat oven 425°F. Coat crust with olive oil.

2. In large nonstick skillet coated with nonstick cooking spray, cook red bell pepper and onion about 5 minutes or until crisp tender. Add garlic, spinach and oregano, stirring only until spinach is wilted.

3. Evenly spoon spinach mixture over crust and top with remaining ingredients. Bake 8–10 minutes, or until cheese is melted and crust is done.

MAKES 8 servings
PREP TIME 10 minutes
COOK TIME 15 minutes

TERRIFIC TIP

Look for whole-wheat pizza crust. Freeze leftover pizza slices and reheat for a make-ahead meal another day.

. . . .

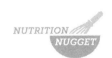
NUTRITION NUGGET

Spinach is a great addition to many dishes because it is concentrated in healthy antioxidant protection.

NUTRITIONAL INFORMATION Calories 199, Calories from Fat 28%, Fat 6 g, Saturated Fat 2 g, Cholesterol 24 mg, Sodium 362 mg, Carbohydrates 21 g, Dietary Fiber 2 g, Total Sugars 2 g, Protein 14 g
DIABETIC EXCHANGES 1 1/2 starch, 1 1/2 lean meat

BLACKENED CHICKEN
WITH AVOCADO CREAM SAUCE

Quick cooking spicy-seasoned chicken with cool avocado sauce makes an unbeatable combination. The blackened chicken may also be served without the sauce.

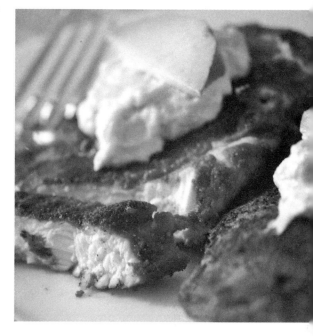

1 1/2 teaspoons paprika
1 1/2 teaspoons cumin
1/4 teaspoon cayenne pepper
1 teaspoon onion powder
Salt and pepper to taste
1 1/2 pounds boneless, skinless chicken breasts
  (4 breasts)

1 In small bowl, mix paprika, cumin, cayenne, onion powder, and season to taste. Coat chicken breasts with mixture.

2 In large nonstick pan coated with nonstick cooking spray, cook chicken over medium-high heat, 5–7 minutes on each side, or until done.

3 Serve topped with Avocado Cream Sauce.

AVOCADO CREAM SAUCE

1/3 cup nonfat plain Greek yogurt
1 avocado, mashed
1 1/2 teaspoons lemon juice
1/2 teaspoon garlic powder

1 In small bowl, mix together all sauce ingredients until creamy.

MAKES 4 servings
PREP TIME 15 minutes
COOK TIME 15 minutes

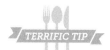
TERRIFIC TIP

Adjust cayenne to your taste preference. The Avocado Cream Sauce also makes a great sandwich spread or dipping sauce.

. . . .

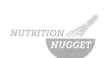
NUTRITION NUGGET

Avocado is a rich source of healthy unsaturated fats that help your body to absorb and use vitamins, as well as helping to maintain cell membranes.

NUTRITIONAL INFORMATION Calories 295, Calories from Fat 37%, Fat 12 g, Saturated Fat 2 g, Cholesterol 110 mg, Sodium 210 mg, Carbohydrates 7 g, Dietary Fiber 4 g, Total Sugars 1 g, Protein 39 g
DIABETIC EXCHANGES 1/2 carbohydrate, 5 lean meat

F

CHICKEN THAI ENCHILADAS

Pick up a rotisserie chicken for this simple Thai-licious enchilada with flavorful chicken filling and a fabulous light coconut-peanut butter sauce.

1/2 cup chopped onion
1/2 cup shredded carrots
1/2 cup shredded cabbage
1 tablespoon minced garlic
2 cups chopped skinless rotisserie chicken
1 bunch green onions, chopped and divided

1/3 cup chopped peanuts
1/4 cup chopped fresh cilantro, optional
1 (13 1/2-ounce) can lite coconut milk, divided
1/2 cup sweet chili sauce, divided
1/4 cup peanut butter
10 flour tortillas

1 Preheat oven 350°F. Coat 13×9×2-inch baking dish with nonstick cooking spray.

2 In large nonstick skillet coated with nonstick cooking spray, stir fry onion, carrots, cabbage, and garlic until almost tender, about 5 minutes.

3 Add chicken, green onions, peanuts, and cilantro, if desired. Add 3/4 cup coconut milk and 1/4 cup sweet chili sauce, mixing to combine.

4 In small bowl, whisk together remaining coconut milk, sweet chili sauce and peanut butter. Pour thin layer of sauce on bottom of dish.

5 Heat tortillas in microwave few seconds to soften, if desired. Place heaping 1/4 cup chicken mixture in each tortilla, roll up, and place seam side down in dish. Spoon remaining coconut milk mixture over enchiladas. Bake 20 minutes. Serve with chopped peanuts and cilantro, if desired

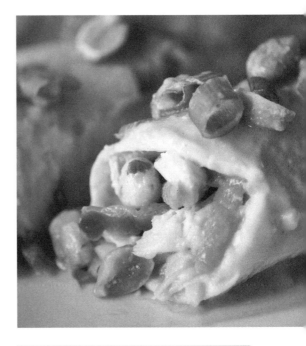

MAKES 10 chicken enchiladas
PREP TIME 20 minutes
COOK TIME 25 minutes

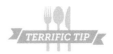

Don't let this recipe intimidate you! Buy pre-shredded cabbage and carrots, a rotisserie chicken and a few cans and you are done!

. . . .

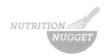

Unlike cow's milk, coconut milk is lactose-free so can be used as a milk substitute by those with lactose intolerance.

NUTRITIONAL INFORMATION Calories 286, Calories from Fat 30%, Fat 9 g, Saturated Fat 3 g, Cholesterol 24 mg, Sodium 599 mg, Carbohydrates 34 g, Dietary Fiber 4 g, Total Sugars 6 g, Protein 16 g
DIABETIC EXCHANGES 2 starch, 1 vegetable, 2 lean meat

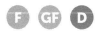

SNAPPY SALMON BURGERS

Fresh salmon makes all the difference with these sensationally delicious burgers full of snap and pop! Serve on a bun or a plate with your favorite condiments.

2 pounds fresh salmon fillets, skinned
1/2 cup chopped green onions
1/2 teaspoon minced garlic
2 tablespoons lemon juice
1/2 teaspoon dried dill weed leaves
Salt and pepper to taste
1 egg
1 egg white
2 cups crisp rice cereal

1 With knife or food processor, chop salmon into small pieces.

2 In large bowl, mix together salmon, green onions, garlic, lemon juice, dill and season to taste.

3 In another bowl, whisk together egg and egg white and add to salmon mixture.

4 Using your hands, gently mix salmon mixture with cereal (mixture will be loose). Form mixture into burgers.

5 Heat large nonstick skillet coated with nonstick cooking spray over medium heat. Cook 3–4 minutes on each side or until golden brown.

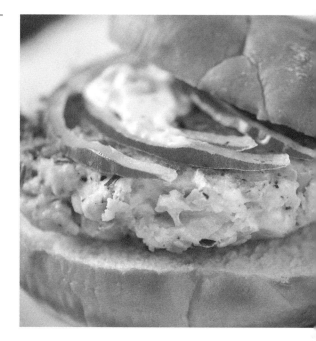

MAKES 8 salmon burgers
PREP TIME 15 minutes
COOK TIME 10 minutes

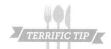
TERRIFIC TIP

Salmon patties may be made ahead and refrigerated until ready to cook. If grilling, place salmon patties in freezer about 20-30 minutes so they'll hold together better. If freezing, freeze before cooking.

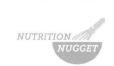
NUTRITION NUGGET

Salmon is an excellent source of omega-3 fatty acids, providing a host of nutritional benefits including reduced risk of heart disease and inflammation.

NUTRITIONAL INFORMATION Calories 188, Calories from Fat 29%, Fat 6 g, Saturated Fat 1 g, Cholesterol 76 mg, Sodium 142 mg, Carbohydrates 7 g, Dietary Fiber 0 g, Total Sugars 1 g, Protein 25 g

DIABETIC EXCHANGES 1/2 starch, 3 lean meat

F **GF** **D**

GLAZED SALMON

Trying to include salmon in your diet? Here's my #1 easy, favorite recipe (went viral on YouTube); rumor is this is the best salmon ever. A delicious glaze covers the seared salmon.

1/4 cup honey
2 tablespoons low-sodium soy sauce
2 tablespoons lime juice
1 tablespoon Dijon mustard
4 (6-ounce) salmon fillets

1 In small bowl, whisk together honey, soy sauce, lime juice, and mustard. Marinate salmon in sauce in refrigerator several hours, or time permitted (do not discard marinade).

2 In nonstick skillet coated with nonstick cooking spray, cook salmon on each side, 3–5 minutes, until golden brown, crispy, and just cooked through. Transfer salmon to platter.

3 Add remaining honey glaze to skillet, and simmer, stirring, until mixture comes to boil. Return salmon to skillet, heat thoroughly, and serve immediately.

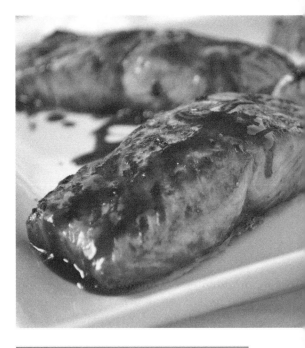

MAKES 4 servings

PREP TIME 5 minutes + time to marinate

COOK TIME 10 minutes

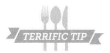
TERRIFIC TIP

Whenever I need to marinate anything, I always use a plastic bag for easy cleanup.

• • • • • • • • • • • • • • • • •

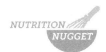
NUTRITION **NUGGET**

Salmon is an excellent source of heart-healthy omega-3 fatty acids and B vitamins as well as vitamins A, D and E.

NUTRITIONAL INFORMATION Calories 297, Calories from Fat 24%, Fat 8 g, Saturated Fat 1 g, Cholesterol 80 mg, Sodium 403 mg, Carbohydrates 20 g, Dietary Fiber 0 g, Total Sugars 19 g, Protein 36 g

DIABETIC EXCHANGES 1 1/2 other carbohydrate, 5 lean meat

SALMON CEVICHE
WITH CUCUMBER AND MANGO

Salmon, cucumber, mango, citrus juices, and fresh ingredients make a delectable heart-healthy dish perfect for a super light meal.

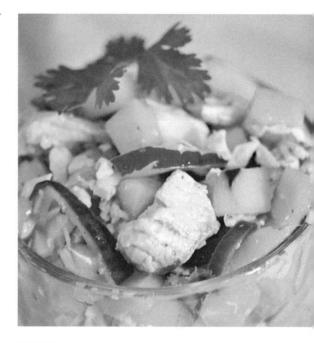

1 1/2 pounds skinless, salmon fillets, cut into 1/2-inch cubes

1/2 teaspoon apple cider vinegar

1 teaspoon olive oil

Juice of 4 limes (about 1/2 cup lime juice)

1/4 cup orange juice

1 mango, peeled, pitted, and diced (about 1 1/2 cups)

1 cucumber, seeded and diced

2 tablespoons finely sliced red onion

1 tablespoon coarsely chopped fresh cilantro

1 thinly sliced jalapeño or to taste

1/2 teaspoon dried oregano leaves

Salt and pepper to taste

1 In medium pot, fill half with water and bring to boil.

2 When water boils, remove from stove, and add salmon cubes to simmering water. Leave salmon in pot, covered, 6 minutes.

3 Remove immediately and transfer to dish. Cool and refrigerate.

4 Meanwhile, in large glass bowl, combine remaining ingredients and season to taste. Gently toss salmon into mango mixture. Refrigerate until serving.

MAKES 8 (3/4-cup) servings

PREP TIME 15 minutes

COOK TIME 6 minutes

TERRIFIC TIP

To seed a cucumber, cut in half and run spoon down the center to easily remove the seeds.

DOC'S NOTE

Salmon is rich in omega-3 fatty acids, having a wide variety of benefits from reducing the risk of heart disease and stroke to reducing joint pain from inflammation—and is better absorbed through food than supplements.

NUTRITIONAL INFORMATION Calories 164, Calories from fat 25%, Fat 5 g, Saturated Fat 1 g, Cholesterol 40 mg, Sodium 67 mg, Carbohydrates 12 g, Dietary Fiber 1 g, Total Sugars 8 g, Protein 19 g

DIABETIC EXCHANGES 1 fruit, 2 1/2 lean meat

OVEN FRIED FISH

Struggling with cooking fish? Try this fish rescue recipe for easy, crunchy fried fish.

2 tablespoons olive oil
2/3 cup buttermilk
Hot sauce to taste
2 teaspoons Dijon mustard
1 teaspoon minced garlic
Salt and pepper to taste
1 1/2 pounds fish fillets
2/3 cup all-purpose flour
2/3 cup yellow cornmeal

1. Preheat oven 475°F. Coat baking pan with olive oil and place pan in oven to heat.

2. In zip-top plastic bag, combine buttermilk, hot sauce, mustard and garlic. Season fish to taste and add to buttermilk mixture. Let sit 15 minutes.

3. In shallow bowl or plate, mix flour and cornmeal together. Remove fish from buttermilk, letting excess drip off, and dredge on both sides with cornmeal mixture. Transfer to hot baking pan.

4. Bake 6 minutes, then carefully turn fish and continue cooking 5 minutes more, or until cooked through and golden.

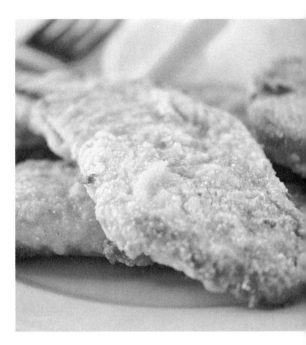

MAKES 6 servings
PREP TIME 20 minutes
COOK TIME 15 minutes

TERRIFIC TIP

The secret trick to crispy fish is to make sure to start with a hot pan.

. . . .

NUTRITION
NUGGET

Fatty fish contain vitamin D, which helps to prevent swelling and soreness.

NUTRITIONAL INFORMATION Calories 173, Calories from Fat 24%, Fat 4 g, Saturated Fat 1 g, Cholesterol 44 mg, Sodium 93 mg, Carbohydrates 13 g, Dietary Fiber 1 g, Total Sugars 1 g, Protein 20 g

DIABETIC EXCHANGES 1 starch, 3 lean meat

FISH TACOS
WITH MANGO PICO

Southwestern seasoned fish topped with a cool Mango Pico makes a mouthwatering light meal.

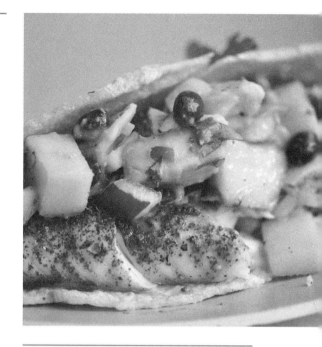

1 pound tilapia fillets, rinsed and patted dry
1 tablespoon olive oil
1 teaspoon chili powder
1/2 teaspoon ground cumin
1/2 teaspoon dried oregano leaves
1/2 teaspoon paprika
Salt and pepper to taste
8 corn tortillas

1 Preheat oven 425°F. Line baking pan with foil and coat with nonstick cooking spray.

2 Place fish on prepared pan. In small bowl, combine oil, chili powder, cumin, oregano, paprika, and season to taste. Spread over fish. Bake 15–18 minutes or until fish flakes with fork.

3 Spray tortillas on each side with nonstick cooking spray and warm tortillas in pan about 1 minute on each side or in microwave about 30 seconds.

4 Divide fish to fill tortillas and top with Mango Pico.

MANGO PICO

2 cups chopped mango
1 tablespoon lime juice
1 tablespoon chopped cilantro
1/4 cup chopped red onion
1 chopped jalapeño or to taste
Salt and pepper to taste

1 In medium bowl, combine all ingredients.

MAKES 4 servings with 1/2 cup mango pico
PREP TIME 15 minutes
COOK TIME 20 minutes

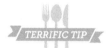
TERRIFIC TIP

You can also add avocado and black beans to the Mango Pico. Don't feel like making Mango Pico, just open a jar of salsa instead.

. . . .

DOC'S NOTE

It is recommended that at least two servings of fish be eaten weekly.

NUTRITIONAL INFORMATION Calories 261, Calories from fat 22%, Fat 7 g, Saturated Fat 1 g, Cholesterol 57 mg, Sodium 117 mg, Carbohydrates 28 g, Dietary Fiber 3 g, Total Sugars 12 g, Protein 25 g
DIABETIC EXCHANGES 1 starch, 1 fruit, 3 lean meat

CRAWFISH ETOUFFEE

This easy-to-follow and healthier version of the popular Louisiana Crawfish Etouffee— Louisiana crawfish simmered with seasonings in a light roux— will be a favorite Cajun recipe. Serve over rice.

2 tablespoons olive oil
3 tablespoons all-purpose flour
1 onion, chopped
1/2 cup chopped green bell pepper
1 teaspoon minced garlic
1 cup fat-free chicken broth
1 tablespoon paprika
1 pound Louisiana crawfish tails, rinsed and drained
Salt and pepper to taste
1 bunch green onions, stems only, finely chopped

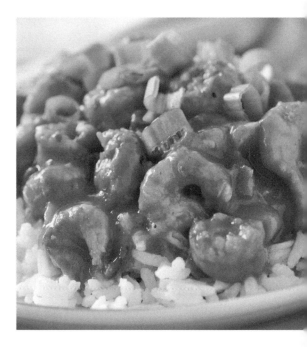

1 In large nonstick skillet coated with nonstick cooking spray, heat oil and stir in flour. Cook over medium heat until light brown, about 6–8 minutes, stirring constantly. Add onion, green pepper, and garlic. Sauté until tender, about 5 minutes.

2 Gradually add broth and stir until thickened. Add paprika and bring to boil, reduce heat, cover, and cook about 5 minutes, stirring occasionally.

3 Add crawfish and continue cooking 5 more minutes or until heated. Season to taste. Stir in green onions before serving.

MAKES 4 (1-cup) servings
PREP TIME 10 minutes
COOK TIME 25–30 minutes

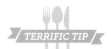
TERRIFIC TIP

The browned flour and oil create a roux that gives the etouffee deep rich flavor.

· · · · · · · · · · · · · · · · ·

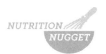
NUTRITION
NUGGET

Try serving with brown rice to easily boost fiber: 1 cup rice equals 1g fiber while 1 cup brown rice equals 3g fiber.

NUTRITIONAL INFORMATION Calories 220, Calories from Fat 36%, Fat 9 g, Saturated Fat 1 g, Cholesterol 155 mg, Sodium 217 mg, Carbohydrates 13 g, Dietary Fiber 4 g, Total Sugars 4 g, Protein 22 g

DIABETIC EXCHANGES 1 carbohydrate, 3 lean meat

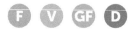

SWEET POTATO CORNBREAD DRESSING

The ultimate holiday dressing combining sweet potatoes and cornbread into one amazing dish.

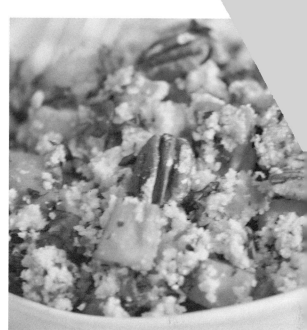

2 tablespoons canola oil
2 cups peeled sweet potato small chunks
1 cup chopped onion
1 cup chopped celery
1/4 cup chopped fresh parsley
1 teaspoon ground ginger
5 cups crumbled cooked cornbread
1/4 cup chopped pecans, toasted
Vegetable broth, as needed

1 Preheat oven 375°F. Coat 3-quart baking dish with nonstick cooking spray.

2 In large nonstick skillet coated with nonstick cooking spray, heat oil over medium heat. Sauté sweet potatoes, onion, and celery 7–10 minutes or until just tender, stirring.

3 Spoon mixture into large mixing bowl. Stir in parsley and ginger. Add cornbread and pecans and toss gently to coat. Add broth to moisten.

4 Place stuffing in prepared dish. Bake, uncovered, 35–45 minutes or until heated through.

MAKES 10 (3/4 cup) servings
PREP TIME 20 minutes
COOK TIME 45–55 minutes

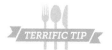

For a short cut, prepare or buy cornbread and toast pecans ahead of time.

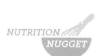

Sweet potatoes are packed with vitamins and enhance the nutritional value of this recipe.

NUTRITIONAL INFORMATION Calories 241, Calories from fat 42%, Fat 9 g, Saturated Fat 1 g, Cholesterol 6 mg, Sodium 332 mg, Carbohydrate 36 g, Dietary Fiber 3 g, Total Sugars 12 g, Protein 4 g

DIABETIC EXCHANGES 2 1/2 starch, 1 1/2 fat

...TED BROCCOLI

...sting broccoli is easy cooking and easy clean up; tossed with olive oil and cheese for a snazzy side. Look for pre-cut broccoli florets in the grocery store for even less prep work.

4 cups broccoli florets
2 tablespoons olive oil
Salt and pepper to taste
2 tablespoons grated Parmesan cheese
1 tablespoons lemon juice
1 teaspoon lemon rind, optional
2 teaspoons pine nuts, toasted, optional

1 Preheat oven 425°F. Line baking pan with foil and coat with nonstick cooking spray.

2 Toss broccoli with olive oil and season to taste; arrange in single layer on pan. Roast about 20 minutes or until tender and browned around edges.

3 Remove from oven and toss with cheese, lemon juice, lemon rind and pine nuts, if desired.

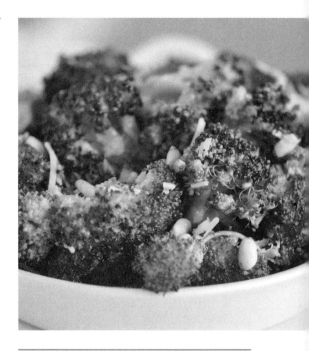

MAKES 6 (2/3-cup) servings
PREP TIME 5 minutes
COOK TIME 20 minutes

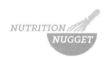
TERRIFIC TIP

If using fresh lemons, you have lemon rind and if not, leave it out and grab bottled lemon juice. Pine nuts or any toasted nut may be used.

. . . .

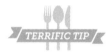
NUTRITION **NUGGET**

Broccoli is an anti-inflammatory powerhouse, rich in antioxidants, vitamin C, and carotenoids.

NUTRITIONAL INFORMATION Calories 68, Calories from Fat 64%, Fat 5 g, Saturated Fat 1 g, Cholesterol 1 mg, Sodium 46 mg, Carbohydrates 4 g, Dietary Fiber 2 g, Total Sugars 1 g, Protein 2 g
DIABETIC EXCHANGES 1 vegetable, 1 fat

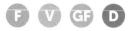

CAULIFLOWER CRISP STIR-FRY

Wait until you try this toasty and tasty simple cauliflower stir-fry!

2 tablespoons olive oil
4 cups cauliflower florets, cut into tiny pieces
Salt and pepper to taste
2 tablespoons grated Parmesan cheese

1 In large nonstick skillet, heat olive oil and add cauliflower, cook, stirring, 6-8 minutes, or until tender and crispy brown on edges.

2 Season to taste. Sprinkle with Parmesan cheese, serve.

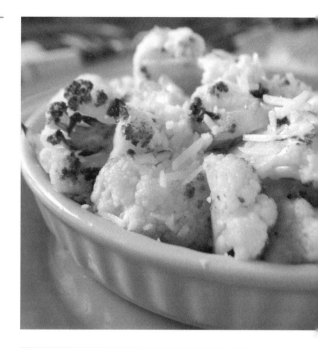

MAKES 4 (3/4 cup) servings
PREP TIME 5 minutes
COOK TIME 8 minutes

TERRIFIC TIP

You can use already cut cauliflower florets but you still want to cut into smaller pieces.

. . . .

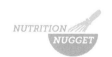

NUTRITION NUGGET

Cauliflower contains immune boosting antioxidants vitamin C and folate.

NUTRITIONAL INFORMATION Calories 97, Calories from fat 67%, Fat 8 g, Saturated Fat 1 g, Cholesterol 2 mg, Sodium 68 mg, Carbohydrate 5 g, Dietary Fiber 2 g, Total Sugars 2 g, Protein 3 g

DIABETIC EXCHANGES 1 vegetable, 1 1/2 fat

SOUTHWESTERN ROASTED VEGETABLES

Jazz up veggies by tossing with taco seasoning and roasting in the oven. Fantastic and uncomplicated! Add your favorite veggies to the mixture.

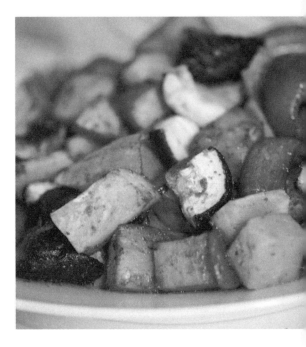

4 cups peeled, cubed sweet potatoes, cut into 1-inch cubes
1 1/2 cups zucchini, cut into small chunks
1 cup quartered red onion slices
3 cups baby portabella mushrooms, quartered
2 tablespoons olive oil
3 tablespoons reduced-sodium taco seasoning mix

1 Preheat oven 425°F. Line baking pan with foil and coat with nonstick cooking spray.

2 On prepared baking pan, toss sweet potatoes, zucchini, onion, and mushrooms with olive oil to coat vegetables. Sprinkle with taco seasoning, toss.

3 Bake 35-40 minutes, turning after 20 minutes, or until vegetables are tender and roasted.

MAKES 8 (1/2-cup) servings
PREP TIME 15 minutes
COOK TIME 40 minutes

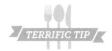

Pop any leftovers into a soup pot with some chicken broth for a terrific Southwestern vegetable soup.

. . . .

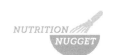

Sweet potato and zucchini are rich in the antioxidant, vitamin A, low in calories and a good source of fiber.

NUTRITIONAL INFORMATION Calories 110, Calories from Fat 31%, Fat 4 g, Saturated Fat 1 g, Cholesterol 0 mg, Sodium 209 mg, Carbohydrates 17 g, Dietary Fiber 3 g, Total Sugars 5 g, Protein 2 g

DIABETIC EXCHANGES 1 starch, 1/2 fat

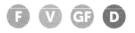

GREEK RICE

Turn rice into a super satisfying rice recipe with spinach and feta.

1 cup brown rice
2 1/4 cups vegetable broth
1 onion, chopped
1 teaspoon minced garlic
2 teaspoons dried oregano leaves
6 cups fresh baby spinach leaves
1/3 cup crumbled feta cheese

1. In nonstick pot, combine rice and broth. Bring to boil, stir, and reduce heat. Cover and simmer 35–45 minutes or until rice is tender.

2. Meanwhile, in large nonstick skillet coated with nonstick cooking spray, sauté onion and garlic until tender. Stir in oregano and spinach, cooking only until spinach wilted. Add cooked rice, mixing well. Sprinkle with cheese.

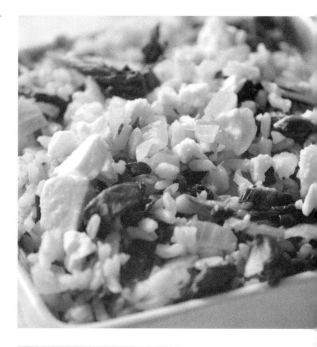

MAKES 6 (2/3 cup) servings
PREP TIME 5 minutes
COOK TIME 45 minutes

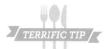

Adjust the onion, mushrooms and feta to your preferences.

· · · · · · · · · · · · · · · · ·

Onions are packed with vitamin C, sulphuric compounds, flavonoids, and phytochemicals which have anticancer properties.

NUTRITIONAL INFORMATION Calories 157, Calories from Fat 16%, Fat 3 g, Saturated Fat 1 g, Cholesterol 8 mg, Sodium 133 mg, Carbohydrates 28 g, Dietary Fiber 3 g, Total Sugars 2 g, Protein 6 g
DIABETIC EXCHANGES 2 starch

QUICK SPANISH RICE

Looking for a quick rice recipe—here you go!

1 (10-ounce) package yellow saffron rice
1 cup salsa
1/3 cup chopped green onions

1 Prepare rice according to package directions.

2 Stir in salsa and green onions.

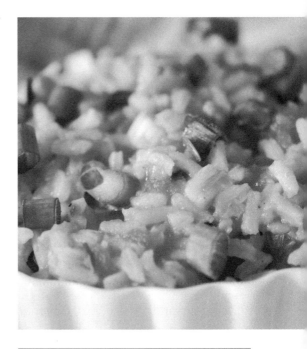

MAKES 8 (1/2-cup) servings

PREP TIME 5 minutes

COOK TIME 20 minutes

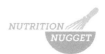

TERRIFIC TIP

Vary the personality of this easy rice with different-flavored salsas.

. . . .

NUTRITION NUGGET

Did you know 1/2 cup salsa = 1 serving vegetables?

NUTRITIONAL INFORMATION Calories 146, Calories from Fat 0, Total Fat 0 g, Saturated Fat 0 g, Cholesterol 0 mg, Sodium 424 mg, Total Carbohydrate 33 g, Dietary Fiber 0 g, Total Sugars 1 g, Protein 3 g

DIABETIC EXCHANGES 2 starch

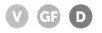

THAI COCONUT RICE MEDLEY
WITH GINGER-PEANUT SAUCE

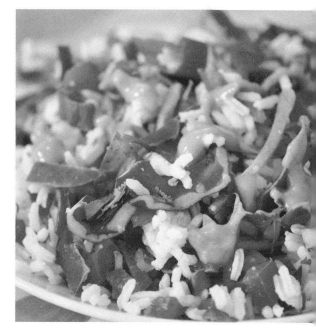

A spectacular mixture of coconut with a vegetable medley and a tangy Ginger Peanut Sauce.

1 1/2 cups jasmine rice	2 cups shredded red cabbage
1 (15-ounce) can lite coconut milk	1 cup shredded carrots
1/2 teaspoon minced garlic	1/2 cup chopped red onion
1 cup water	1/2 cup chopped cilantro
1 red bell pepper, cored and chopped	1/2 cup chopped green onions

1. In medium pot, mix together rice, coconut milk, garlic, and water. Cook according to package directions.

2. In bowl, combine remaining ingredients. When rice is done, fluff with fork and add chopped vegetables.

4. Serve rice medley drizzled with Ginger-Peanut Sauce.

GINGER PEANUT SAUCE

1/3 cup peanut butter	1 teaspoon ground ginger or 3 teaspoons freshly grated ginger
2 tablespoons honey	
2 tablespoons rice vinegar	2 teaspoon sesame oil

1. In small, microwave-safe bowl, combine peanut butter and honey; microwave 15 seconds, or until peanut butter thins. Stir in remaining ingredients; thin with water to desired consistency.

MAKES 10 (1-cup) servings

PREP TIME 20 minutes

COOK TIME 20 minutes

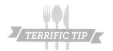

For a hearty entrée, add shredded rotisserie chicken or top with Glazed Salmon (page 184). Make a wrap from the rice!

Coconut milk is dairy, lactose, soy and nut free, making it a good option for those allergic to dairy and nuts.

RICE MEDLEY NUTRITIONAL INFORMATION Calories 140, Calories from Fat 15%, Fat 2 g, Saturated Fat 1 g, Cholesterol 0 mg, Sodium 30 mg, Carbohydrates 27 g, Dietary Fiber 2 g, Total Sugars 3 g, Protein 2 g

DIABETIC EXCHANGES 1 1/2 starch, 1 vegetable

GINGER PEANUT SAUCE NUTRITIONAL INFORMATION Calories 73, Calories from Fat 61%, Fat 5 g, Saturated Fat 1 g, Cholesterol 0 mg, Sodium 41 mg, Carbohydrates 5 g, Dietary Fiber 1 g, Total Sugars 4 g, Protein 2 g

DIABETIC EXCHANGES 1/2 starch, 1 fat

V D

PEACH CRISP

Use fresh or frozen peaches for this luscious cobbler with an oatmeal crumbly topping. So good and comforting hot out of the oven with frozen vanilla yogurt.

1 (16-ounce) package frozen peaches, thawed
1 tablespoons cornstarch
2 tablespoons sugar
1 1/2 teaspoons ground cinnamon, divided
2 tablespoons light brown sugar
1 cup old-fashioned oatmeal
1/2 cup all-purpose flour
2 tablespoons canola oil
2–3 tablespoons orange juice
1 teaspoon vanilla extract

1 Preheat oven 350°F. Coat 2-quart oblong baking dish with nonstick cooking spray.

2 In large bowl, toss together peaches, cornstarch, sugar and 1/2 teaspoon cinnamon. Transfer to prepared dish.

3 In another bowl, mix together brown sugar, oatmeal, flour and remaining 1 teaspoon cinnamon. Stir in oil, orange juice and vanilla until crumbly. Sprinkle on top peaches.

4 Bake 35–40 minutes, or until topping is brown and mixture is bubbly. Serve immediately or refrigerate leftovers.

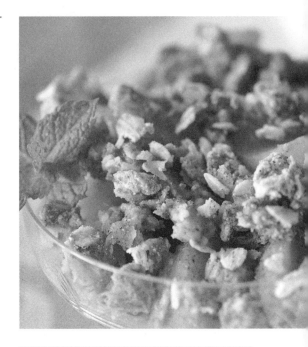

MAKES 6 (1/2 cup) servings
PREP TIME 15 minutes
COOK TIME 35–40 minutes

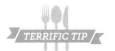
TERRIFIC TIP

Any fruit, fresh or frozen, may be substituted for peaches.

. . . .

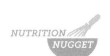
NUTRITION
NUGGET

This dessert is a good source of fiber.

NUTRITIONAL INFORMATION Calories 206, Calories from Fat 27%, Fat 6 g, Saturated Fat 1 g, Cholesterol 0 mg, Sodium 2 mg, Carbohydrates 35 g, Dietary Fiber 4 g, Total Sugars 13 g, Protein 3 g
DIABETIC EXCHANGES 1 starch, 1/2 fruit, 1 other carbohydrate, 1 fat

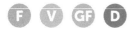

PEANUT BUTTER COOKIES

Yes, these simple ingredients create my favorite peanut butter cookie ever! Believe it or not, there is no flour in this recipe.

1 cup crunchy peanut butter
1/2 cup light brown sugar
1 egg
1/2 teaspoon baking soda
1/4 cup chopped peanuts

1 Preheat oven 350°F. Coat baking pan with nonstick cooking spray.

2 In large bowl, combine peanut butter, brown sugar, egg, and baking soda until well combined. Stir in peanuts.

3 Place dough by teaspoonfuls on nonstick baking pan and press down with a fork to form ridges. Bake 10–12 minutes or until lightly browned.

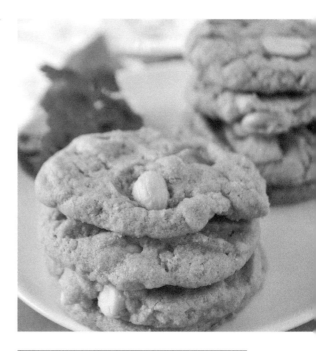

MAKES 30 cookies
PREP TIME 15 minutes
COOK TIME 10–12 minutes

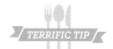

Use a lightly floured fork to keep it from sticking to the cookie batter when you make ridges in the cookies. Don't use a floured fork for gluten-free.

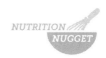

Keep these in the freezer for a quick diabetic-friendly sweet treat.

NUTRITIONAL INFORMATION Calories 73, Calories from Fat 57%, Fat 5 g, Saturated Fat 1 g, Cholesterol 6 mg, Sodium 59 mg, Carbohydrates 6 g, Dietary Fiber 1 g, Total Sugars 4 g, Protein 3 g

DIABETIC EXCHANGES 1/2 other carbohydrate, 1 fat

INDEX

· ·